Advances in Anatomy, Embryology and Cell Biology
Ergebnisse der Anatomie und Entwicklungsgeschichte
Revues d'anatomie et de morphologie expérimentale

Vol. 55 · Fasc. 5

The Advances publishes reviews and critical articles covering the entire field of normal anatomy (cytology, histology, cyto- and histochemistry, electron microscopy, macroscopy, experimental morphology and embryology and comparative anatomy). Papers dealing with anthropology and clinical morphology will also be accepted with the aim of encouraging co-operation between anatomy and related disciplines.

Papers, which may be in English, French or German, are normally commissioned, but original papers and communications may be submitted and will be considered so long as they deal with a subject comprehensively and meet the requirements of the "Advances".

For speed of publication and breadth of distribution, this journal appears in single issues which can be purchased separately; 6 issues constitute one volume.

It is a fundamental condition that submitted manuscripts have not been, and will not simultaneously be submitted or published elsewhere. With the acceptance of a manuscript for publication, the publisher acquires full and exclusive copyright for all languages and countries. 25 copies of each paper are supplied free of charge.

Die Ergebnisse dienen der Veröffentlichung zusammenfassender und kritischer Artikel aus dem Gesamtgebiet der normalen Anatomie (Cytologie, Histologie, Cyto- und Histochemie, Elektronenmikroskopie, Makroskopie, experimentelle Morphologie und Embryologie und vergleichende Anatomie). Aufgenommen werden ferner Arbeiten anthropologischen und morphologisch-klinischen Inhalts, mit dem Ziel, die Zusammenarbeit zwischen Anatomie und Nachbardisziplinen zu fördern.

Zur Veröffentlichung gelangen in erster Linie angeforderte Manuskripte, jedoch werden auch eingesandte Arbeiten und Originalmitteilungen berücksichtigt, sofern sie ein Gebiet umfassend abhandeln und den Anforderungen der „Ergebnisse" genügen. Die Veröffentlichungen erfolgen in englischer, deutscher oder französischer Sprache.

Die Arbeiten erscheinen im Interesse einer raschen Veröffentlichung und einer weiten Verbreitung als einzeln berechnete Hefte; je 6 Hefte bilden einen Band.

Grundsätzlich dürfen nur Arbeiten eingesandt werden, die nicht gleichzeitig an anderer Stelle zur Veröffentlichung eingereicht oder bereits veröffentlicht worden sind. Der Autor verpflichtet sich, seinen Beitrag auch nachträglich nicht an anderer Stelle zu publizieren. Die Mitarbeiter erhalten von ihren Arbeiten zusammen 25 Freiexemplare.

Les résultats publient des sommaires et des articles critiques concernant l'ensemble du domaine de l'anatomie normale (cytologie, histologie, cyto- et histochimie, microscopie électronique, macroscopie, morphologie expérimentale, embryologie et anatomie comparée). Seront publiés en outre les articles traitant de l'anthropologie et de la morphologie clinique, en vue d'encourager la collaboration entre l'anatomie et les disciplines voisines.

Seront publiés en priorité les articles expressément demandés, nous tiendrons toutefois compte des articles qui nous seront envoyés dans la mesure où ils traitent d'un sejet dans son ensemble et correspondent aux standards des « Revues ». Les publications seront faites en langues anglaise, allemande ou française.

Dans l'intérêt d'une publication rapide et d'une large diffusion les travaux publiés paraitront dans des cahiers individuels, diffusés séparément: 6 cahiers forment un volume.

En principe, seuls les manuscripts qui n'ont encore été publiés ni dans le pays d'origine ni à l'étranger peuvent nous être soumis. L'auteur s'engage en outre à ne pas les publier ailleurs ultérieurement. Les auteurs recevront 25 exemplaires gratuits de leur publication.

**Manuscripts should be addressed to / Manuskripte sind zu senden an / Envoyer les manuscrits à:**

Prof. Dr. A. BRODAL, Universitetet i Oslo, Anatomisk Institutt, Karl Johans Gate 47 (Domus Media), Oslo 1 / Norwegen

Prof. W. HILD, Department of Anatomy, Medical Branch, The University of Texas, Galveston, Texas 77550/USA

Prof. Dr. J. van LIMBORGH, Universiteit van Amsterdam, Anatomisch-Embryologisch Laboratorium, Mauritskade 61, Amsterdam-O/Holland

Prof. Dr. R. ORTMANN, Anatomisches Institut der Universität, Lindenburg, D-5000 Köln-Lindenthal

Prof. Dr. T. H. SCHIEBLER, Anatomisches Institut der Universität, Koellikerstraße 6, D-8700 Würzburg

Prof. Dr. G. TÖNDURY, Direktion der Anatomie, Gloriastraße 19, CH-8006 Zürich/Schweiz

Prof. Dr. E. WOLFF, Lab. d'Embryologie Experimentale, College de France, 11 Place Marcelin Berthelot, F-75005 Paris/Frankreich

Gerald Fleischer

# Evolutionary Principles
# of the Mammalian Middle Ear

With 25 Figures

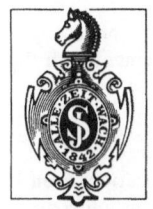

Springer-Verlag Berlin Heidelberg New York 1978

Dr. Gerald Fleischer, c/o Umweltbundesamt, Bismarckplatz 1, D-1000 Berlin 33

Habilitations-Schrift at the School of Medicine, Justus-Liebig-University, Giessen, Federal Republic of Germany

ISBN-13: 978-3-540-09140-0        e-ISBN-13: 978-3-642-67143-2
DOI: 10.1007/978-3-642-67143-2

Composition, printing and binding: H. Stürtz AG, Universitätsdruckerei, Würzburg
2121/3321-543210

# Contents

# Symbols

◉   tympanic  membrane

◗   tympanic  plate

▮   malleus

◭   stapes

●   center  of  mass

★   insertion  of  the
tensor  tympani  muscle

▰▷   elastic  element

✳   cochlea

Pe   periotic  bone

Ty   tympanic  bone

Common symbols used in the figures
*Note:* All figures show the left ear

6

# 1. Introduction and Scope

Mammals are a highly successful group of animals in that they have conquered even the most hostile environments and developed impressive specializations in the process. Some, like the shrews *Suncus* or *Crocidura*, weigh only a few grams and are thus smaller than the largest insects. The whales, on the other hand, are millions of times more massive, the blue whale, *Balaenoptera musculus*, reaching a weight of 100 metric tons and more. Some species, like the Bathyergidae, stay below the ground throughout their life, while others live in the desert, or climb in the mountains, wade through swamps, or even venture out into the open sea without ever returning to the shore. *Petaurus, Cynocephalus,* as well as a variety of others are gliders and the Chiroptera are all highly skilled flyers, while others, like the antarctic Weddell seal, *Leptonychotes*, spend most of their time near or under the ice, diving for food. The bats use a sophisticated echo-location system, based on the emission an reception of ultrasonic sounds, as do the dolphins. Mysticetes are capable of communicating over large distances using very low frequences. Last but not least, man owes much of his superiority to the development of language.

In contrast to this tremendous diversity in size, environment, and physiologic capabilities, the mammalian middle ear appears rather conservative. Although the configuration of its components differs to a great extent, nevertheless the morphology is basically the same throughout the mammals: the tympanic bone, the three auditory ossicles, the two middle ear muscles, and the tympanic membrane or its bony equivalent in some odontocetes. The middle ear cavity is filled with air, regardless of whether the animal is terrestrial or aquatic.

Much work has been devoted to the structure of the middle ear, and especially in the last quarter century, much has been learned as to the hearing capabilities of mammals. The theory of hearing is now a complex specialty, but most of its research is performed on only a few species such as cats, guinea pigs, rabbits, and the squirrel monkey, *Saimiri*. Man and some bats have also been examined in detail. A review of the immense literature on the mammalian ear will not be attempted. Instead a unifying concept will be presented attempting to explain the evolutionary radiation of the mammalian middle ear as a function of the hearing capability, the size of the sound-conducting apparatus, and the environment. The envisaged coverage of the entire range of mammals, of necessity excludes a detailed discussion of many individual species. Moreover, it will be necessary to group a variety of similar ears according to certain types, in order to demonstrate the general principles more clearly.

Over the last decade the author has studied the ears of more than 300 species of mammals, from the tiny insectivores to the blue whale, man included. Members of all orders and suborders have been examined; only a few, rare families of mammals have not been scrutinized thus far. Most of this work has been published. If not mentioned otherwise the various morphologic observations and statements are based on the work of the author. Basic mechanisms of acoustics and of mechanical vibrations are used to illuminate the underlying principles of the evolutionary changes.

A number of concepts on the middle ear have been published, but they are based on "normal" species, cats or guinea pigs, and do not attempt to explain the evolution of the ear. Undoubtedly one reason for this omission is simply the fact that the ears of the highly specialized forms, dolphins, whales, and to some extent the extremely small mammals, have not been known well enough to develop a unifying concept of the middle ear for all mammals. The present paper gives an initial approximation of the parameters involved and how they affected the course of the middle ear's evolution. Since predictions are made as to physical properties such as mass, distribution of mass, and stiffness of some structures as related to hearing capability, the validity of many statements can be tested experimentally. It is hoped that the study will contribute to the fledgling field of theoretical morphology of the ear.

## 2. The Ancestral Middle Ear

The transition from the reptilian to the mammalian stage of the otic region will not be discussed here. Of interest within the scope of this paper is the evolution of the middle ear apparatus after a truly mammalian condition had already developed. The latter is characterized by the incorporation into the middle ear of malleus, incus, and the tympanic bone. Both the monotremes as well as the therians (marsupials plus placentals) seem to have arrived at the mammalian stage independently. Since the ear of the monotremes is not a typically mammalian one and did not evolve very much it shall be mentioned only briefly. More details can be found in Fleischer (1973a).

The original middle ear, common to marsupials and placentals, is a rather primitive arrangement (Fig. 1). The tympanic membrane is held by the tympanic bone, which forms a ring with a missing segment. Connective tissue alone holds the tympanic bone in place, a condition still found among insectivores and marsupials (and in *Ornithorhynchus*). The malleus, the main components of which are the transversal part and the manubrium attached to it, has an unfamiliar shape. Malleus and tympanic bone are connected via the gonial, a bony element fused to both. Hence the malleus seems more or less immobile. Riding atop the small articulation of the malleus is the incus, its long arm connected to the head of the stapes and its short arm attached to the periotic bone and thus to the skull. The attachment of the incus to the periotic is the major connection between the skull and the middle ear and thus this point very linkely served as hinge for the gradual evolutionary shift of the malleus, gonial, and tympanic bone away from the lower jaw and toward the base of the skull. The stapes is fitted into the oval window of the periotic, exactly as the columella in reptiles. Each ear has two middle ear muscles. The stapedial muscle is attached to the head of the stapes, or at least near to it, while the tensor tympani muscle is attached near the end of the transversal part of the malleus (*pentagon* in Fig. 1). A flaccid part of the tympanic membrane is present, but it is of no further interest.

Although such a middle ear seems rather crude, it nevertheless possesses all essential components. The tympanic membrane serves as a reception area for the sound. Since the tympanic bone, as well as its peripheral connective tissue, is mass loaded by soft tissues, only the thin tympanic membrane is free to vibrate easily due to the air of the outer acoustic meatus on one side and the air of the middle ear cavity on the other. The ancestral ear comprises a mechanical system for transmitting the vibrations of the tympanic membrane to the inner ear. This system effects an increase of the pressure at

## the ancestral middle ear

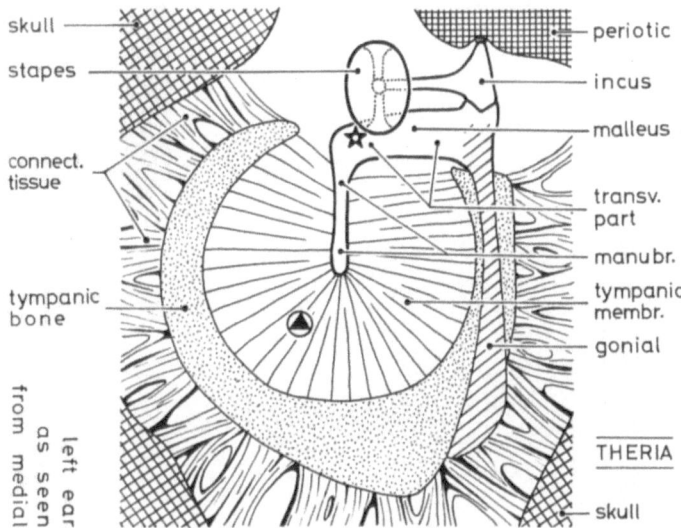

Fig. 1. Semi-schematic view of an ancestral type of the mammalian middle ear, after removal of the cochlea and as seen from the side of the brain. Pars flaccida of the tympanic membrane omitted. Rostral to the lower right. All the following ears are oriented in a similarly standardized way with the manubrium of the malleus in an upright position

the stapedial end compared to that on the tympanic membrane. Most of this increase in pressure is due to the smaller area of the footplate of the stapes when compared to the area of the tympanic membrane, as shown in Fig. 2. The remainder stems from the lever ratio, L1/L2. Such an amplification of the pressure is necessary in order to match the impedance of the air with that of the liquid in the inner ear. Both middle ear muscles, the tensor tympani as well as the stapedius, also allow a certain control of the vibration of the ossicular chain.

While this basic ear is sufficient for a good sense of hearing, it has its shortcomings. Most troublesome is the fact that the middle ear cavity is not surrounded by a rigid wall, but to a great extent by soft connective tissues. Because of this motions within the head – chewing, swallowing, licking, etc. – will cause slight deformations of the middle ear cavity. This in turn alters the pressure inside and thus changes the sensitivity of the ear. Moreover, this may also alter the stiffness of the ossicular chain with equally undesirable effects. The disturbances mentioned are all at low frequencies, so that a high-frequency ear might not be too affected. Development of a low-frequency ear, however, will be seriously hampered by this unstable cavity wall. Therefore it is not surprising to see that nearly all groups of mammals have developed a closed middle ear cavity in one way or another. From the point of hearing, it is unimportant whether or not this bony cavity wall is formed by the tympanic bone or by a combination of other bony elements. In most cases the U-shape tympanic bone was attached to the periotic at both free ends and then it grew in a rostral, occipital, and ventromedial direction in the course of the evolution until it enclosed the middle ear cavity.

Another evolutionary problem is related to the blood supply of the brain in general and to the stapedial artery in particular. Originally the main blood supply of the brain was delivered by the stapedial artery, which runs through the crura of the stapes. This

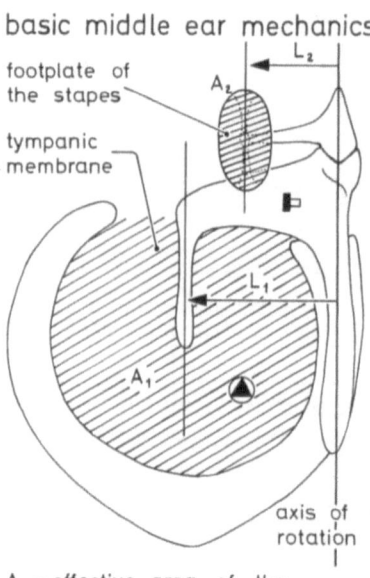

basic middle ear mechanics

footplate of the stapes

tympanic membrane

$L_2$

$A_2$

$L_1$

$A_1$

axis of rotation

$A_1$ = effective area of the tympanic membrane

$A_2$ = area of the footplate

pressure amplification : $R = \dfrac{A_1 \times L_1}{A_2 \times L_2}$

Fig. 2. The basic functional principle of the mammalian middle ear shown for the ancestral type. In addition to this static relation it is also necessary to consider the dynamic response of the sound-conducting apparatus

was possible only because mammals began as small animals. Since the cross section of a blood vessel increases at least with the volume of the tissues to be nourished whereas the stapes increases only slightly with the weight of the animal, such a stapedial artery is not possible in larger mammals. The opening between the crura of the stapes is simply far too narrow in such cases. So the blood supply in the head has to be extensively re-routed as soon as the animals phylogenetically increase their size. The various solutions are described in Tandler (1898, 1902). Hearing is also affected by the pulsation of the artery, especially in ears sensitive to lower frequencies. To reduce this undesirable noise the stapedial artery is surrounded by a bony canal in many small species. The bony canal exists only in that portion of the artery passing through the middle ear. Great care is taken that the bony canal does not touch the stapes when it passes between its crura. While many small mammals have a persistent stapedial artery, rudiments of the latter are found in only a few of the larger species. Some also have a stapedial artery without the bony canal, which poses no disadvantage if either the artery is vestigial or the ear, insensitive to the low frequencies of the noise from the blood flow.

As previously mentioned, mammals began as small creatures with a simple middle ear. This ear then had — and still does — enormous evolutionary potential and modifications of its components permitted the development of the entire variety of hearing organs and hearing capabilities found among mammals.

# 3. Hearing Organ and Skull

Before dealing with the various components of the middle ear, the entire hearing organ is considered. Basically the ear is a microphone and as such it functions quite independent of the head. Of course, the ear has to be provided with space, and with blood, etc., and it is also necessary that the auditory nerve enters the brain, but otherwise the ear is a remarkably independent mechanical arrangement. The fact that mammals have two ears enables them to compare the output from both. In this way a high spatial resolution can be achieved, especially by using the time delay of the arrival of an acoustic signal at each ear. Hence a sound source can be localized much more precisely by two independent ears than is possible with only one ear. The crucial point is that the two ears — or the two microphones used for localization — are independent of each other.

Because the middle ear is a mechanical apparatus it is sensitive to mechanical disturbances, especially to vibrations of the skull. Unfortunately many activities of mammals are accompanied by vibrations of the skull: chewing, especially gnawing, vocalizing, burrowing with the head, fighting with horns and antlers, and many more. If these ear-disturbing activities are reasonably rare, it may simply be sufficient to stop doing them when the animal wants to concentrate on some acoustic signals. In cases where the very life style of the animal entails more or less permanent vibrations of the skull, such behavioral solutions become ineffective and nature obviously seeks to replace them with technical means. Many rodents gnaw extensively over prolonged periods of time but they nevertheless have to be alert to acoustic warnings. Bats and dolphins constantly emit echo-location signals and the mysticete whales occasionally produce songs for hours. Manatees are also persistent singers. Under these circumstances it is desirable to isolate the ear from the vibrations of the skull as much as possible, in order to reduce the mechanical noise. Since both ears pick up the vibrations of the skull, the ears are no longer as independent as is required for good localization without protective measures.

In most mammals, man included, the middle ear cavity has a bony wall and the entire hearing organ is integrated into the skull, as shown on the left side of Fig. 3. The bones are fused with each other and the entire construction is rigid and immobile, relative to the skull. Such a simple arrangement is adequate if vibrations of the skull occur only occasionally. Because of their extensive gnawing activities however, many rodents have a partially isolated ear. Either tympanic or periotic or both expand so that the hearing organ forms a bony shell without incorporating elements of the skull. This bony capsule is connected to the skull via bridges of cartilage, as shown on the right-hand side of Fig. 3. Although certainly not ideal, some isolation will occur, especially at higher frequencies. The common rat (*Rattus*) has such a connection, as do the many voles (*Microtus* and others) and, very impressively for a rodent, the capybara (*Hydrochoerus*). Some of the extreme burrowing species that never venture above the ground may do without such isolation of their ears, because hearing is not that critical to their way of life.

Vocalization can also be the cause for vibrations of the skull, particularly if it is powerful. Bats constantly emit echolocation signals and among them the Rhinolophidae and Hipposideridae are known to produce great sound levels. Especially in these two groups the hearing organ is excellently isolated from the skull. Whereas the cochlea is quite voluminous, the middle ear cavity is very small. Therefor the optical im-

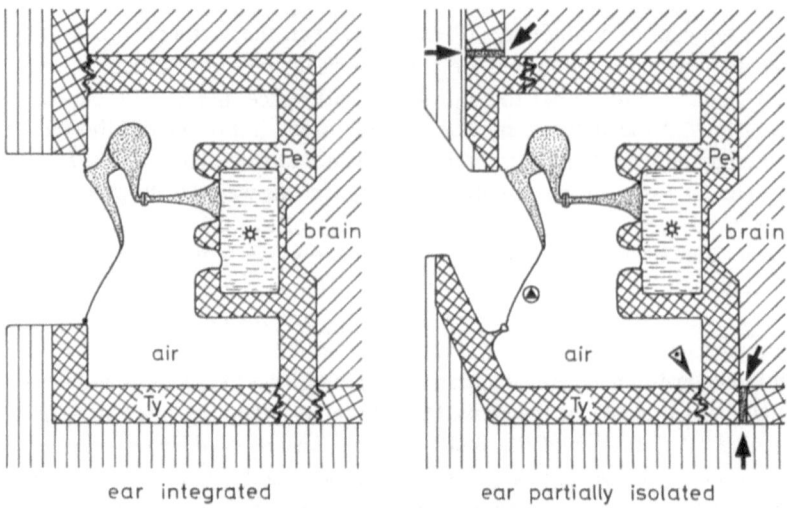

ear integrated                    ear partially isolated

Fig. 3. Two schematic forms of connections between hearing organ and skull in terrestrial species. On the *left* the ear is an integral part of the skull; on the *right* the ear is partially decoupled from the skull. In the latter case the ear is to some extent protected against vibrations of the skull because of intercalated soft-tissue connections (black arrows). The other arrow on the right points toward equivalent structures in Figs. 3 and 4

pression is rather different from the one on the right-hand side of Fig. 3, although the basic principle is the same. Echolocation in these animals abviously requires a precise localization of a sound source (or echo). As mentioned above, this isolation makes the ears independent of each other and protects them from the inevitable vibrations of the skull.

Even more troublesome is the case of an accurate sense of hearing under water, the main reason being that the impedance of water and of soft tissues (fat, muscles, etc.) is very much the same. Therefore sound enters the head essentially unattenuated and the first obstacle in its path is the skull, which reflects some of the acoustic energy. During this process some of the energy will cause the skull to vibrate, thus offsetting or reducing the ears ability to detect time differences of the arrival of a signal. This is one of the reasons why man has such poor ability to localize a sound source under water (Hamilton, 1957; Andersen and Christensen, 1969; Hollien, 1973; Feinstein, 1973; and others). Especially if the diver produces some sound of his own, the directionality of hearing is lost.

Animals using echo location under water must have ears isolated from the skull. It is not surprising that dolphins have ears perfectly isolated from the skull, a fact described and emphasized many times: Boenninghaus (1904), Yamada (1953), Reysenbach de Haan (1957), Fraser and Purves (1960), Purves (1966), and Fleischer (1973b, 1975), to name only a few. The isolation of the hearing organ in the mysticetes is sometimes not that obvious, although it is also well developed. A schematic cross section of the cetacean otic region is shown in Fig. 4. The first impression is that both periotic and tympanic are extremely dense and heavy. Particularly the periotic is much more voluminous than necessary to house the inner ear. Dolphins have a three-dimensional system of

12

## relation between hearing organ and skull

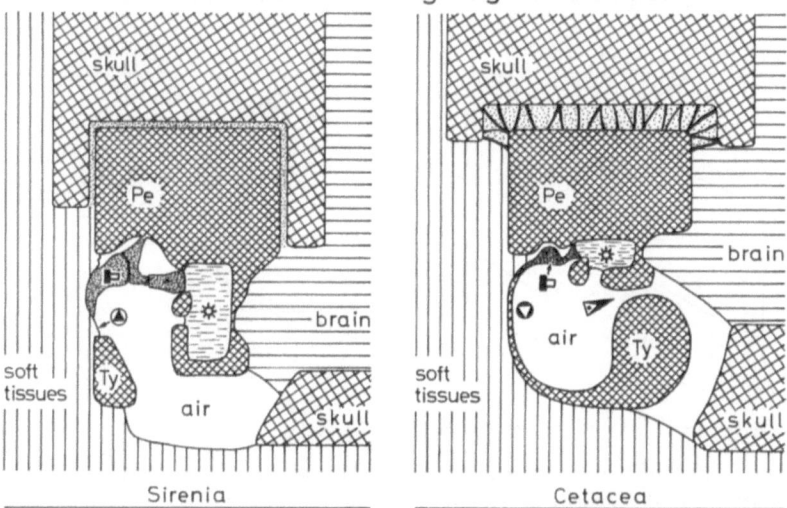

Fig. 4. In cetaceans and sirenians the hearing organ is optimally isolated from the skull. The isolation, which favors a good directionality of hearing, is particularly effective because the periotic bone is very massive and composed of extremely dense bone. No outer acoustic meatus is necessary for hearing under water

ligaments holding the hearing organ in place. Furthermore, an extensive system of soft-walled and air-filled cavities surround the ear except for the lateral wall. There a fat body is in intimate contact with the hearing organ. That the outer acoustic meatus is vestigial is understandable, since its soft tissues are "acoustically transparent". This elaborate suspension and the denseness and compactness of the hearing organ itself effectively protect the ear against vibrations of the skull. No principal difference between the ears of mysticetes and odontocetes can be observed, although the periotic in mysticetes is much more rugged and irregular in shape than it is in odontocetes.

At first glace the hearing organ in the sirenians differs radically from that in cetaceans. However, closer inspection reveals little difference. Again the entire bony hearing organ is impressively dense and heavy and the periotic is much larger that the inner ear (Fig. 4). The squamosal has a concave cavity within which the periotic is fitted. Both are separated by a layer of cartilage. As in the cetaceans the middle ear cavity is filled with air. Manatees have a large tympanic membrane that is tough and bulges outward by the manubrium of the malleus. The tympanic bone is still u-shaped, as in the ancestral ear, but both ends of the u are fused with the periotic. Figure 5 shows the relation between both elements more clearly.

In a "regular" mammal the hearing organ is attached to the skull and because the head is very massive when compared to the ear, the ears are stabilized. In cetaceans and sirenians, on the other hand, the ear is decoupled from the skull and thus the problem of its stabilization arises. This is solved by adding mass to the hearing organ, particularly to the periotic bone. The entire ear in these animals is essentially a mass-spring system, the spring being the soft-tissue connections between the hearing organ and the skull. Such a system is more stable, the more mass is included; and that seems to be the reason why the low-frequency ears of the mysticetes are so extraordinarily heavy, one ear weighing up to several kilograms.

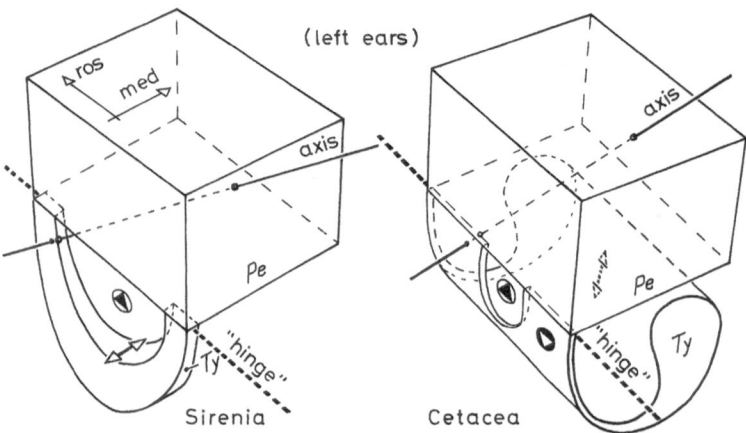

Fig. 5. Relation between periotic bone and tympanic bone in cetaceans and sirenians. The *axis* refers to the rotational axis of the malleus-incus complex, as shown in Figs. 12 and 17. In both groups the tympanic is free to vibrate relative to the periotic. *ros:* rostral; *med:* medial. The *"hinge"* serves only to visualize the vibrational mode of the tympanic bone

Another interesting feature must be considered in connection with Fig. 4 and 5, the relation between periotic and tympanic. Looking first at the sirenians, we see that the tympanic is still a u-shape element fused with the periotic at both ends (Fig. 5). In between lies the tympanic membrane. From Fig. 4 we know liquid or liquid-like soft tissue is outside the tympanic membrane, while on the other side is the air of the middle ear. At such a liquid-air interface sound will be reflected, but some will cause the tympanic membrane and the tympanic bone to vibrate. This is an important mechanism for such an ear: the tympanic bone will vibrate like a tuning fork, relative to the heavy mass of the periotic. Theoretically such a motion of the tympanic is also present in the ancestral ear, but it is certainly not important because sound is mostly reflected from the surface of a terrestrial animal. It is important, however, in sirenians — and in cetaceans — because sound can easily penetrate the soft tissues under water.

At first glance the relation between periotic and tympanic in cetaceans seems to be somewhat different from the situation found in sirenians (Fig. 4). A three-dimensional schematic presentation (Fig. 5) reveals a similarity between both types. In the middle is the tympanic membrane, which is not very large, at least in the dolphins. Rostral and occipital, the tympanic bone is in contact with the periotic. In the mysticetes both of these contacts are true bony fusions while in many, if not in most dolphins, an intimate contact between tympanic and periotic exists but without a fusion of the bones. The actual configuration of these contacts differs to a great extent among the various species. The rostral one, however, is always weaker than the occipital one. While these differences are obvious, important in all of these ears is that the tympanic bone be free to make hingelike motions relative to the periotic, just as it is in the sirenians.

A peculiarity in all cetaceans is the medial rim of the tympanic which is rolled upward and enlarged to a bulky an massive bulge of dense bony material. In all of them this rim remains separate from the periotic bone, i. e. no medial contact between tympanic and periotic is found in any of the cetaceans. This relation is functionally important because it shows that the tympanic is free to "hinge" relative to the periotic along the *dotted line* in Fig. 5. The two other axes shown indicate the rotational axis of the malleus-incus complex, a topic to be discussed later. Because the tympanic is fused with the periotic in sirenians it is obviously no true hingelike motion, but rather a flexion as in a tuning fork. The *interrupted lines* are used only to aid in visualizing the vibrations. Cetaceans also possess a flexional motion between tympanic and periotic.

Since the ears in these marine mammals are not fused with the skull, all the relative motions within the ear have to have a reference mass. That is another reason why the periotic is so large and massive and composed of extremely dense bone. Usually the periotic is much more massive than the tympanic, but there are some exceptions, such as in the pygmy sperm whale (*Kogia*).

Structures like the tympanic-periotic complex have a natural frequency that depends on both the stiffness of the connection between both elements and the distribution of the mass of the tympanic. The periotic will be considered immobile because of its mass. This fundamental natural frequency increases if the stiffness of the connection increases and decreases if the center of mass is shifted away from what was called the "hinge."

Both sirenians and cetaceans have a tympanic bone with a highly characteristic mass distribution. Although the configuration is dissimilar the bulk of the mass of the tympanic is far from the "hinge" in both groups, as seen in Fig. 5. The tympanic is ventrally enlarged in the sirenians, while the cetaceans have the ventromedial bulge. The differences between the various species need not be emphasized but due to these differences a fixed relation cannot be given for all of them. Important is the conclusion, however, that the natural frequency of this arrangement is different in different species, because stiffness and mass distribution are not constant. In other words, this somewhat curious configuration must be seen as the morphologic expression of the construction's vibrational properties. Nature achieved the desired dynamic behavior by shaping it this way.

This digression on the periotic-tympanic complex within this chapter seems justified, because it should be seen in connection with the ears' isolation from the skull. If the periotic-tympanic were not supposed to vibrate relative to each other, cetaceans and sirenians would enclose the middle ear with a thick and massive wall that would be entirely fused. This could be easily done, since mass is no problem in these heavy aquatic mammals.

Seals may appear to be adapted in a similar way to the two groups discussed, but this is not the case. Their ears are only partially isolated from the skull, although the cochlear portion of the periotic remains somewhat separate from the tympanic bone. Since the structure of seal ears has been described by Repenning (1972) more details will not be discussed here.

# 4. Volume of the Middle Ear Cavity

If we consider those middle ears with a bony wall, the structure can be simplified (Fig. 6). Basically a rigid wall and a membrane enclose a certain volume of air. A connection between the volume inside and outside equalizes differences in static pressure. In mammals this connection is the Eustachian tube; in technical systems, e. g., condenser mi-

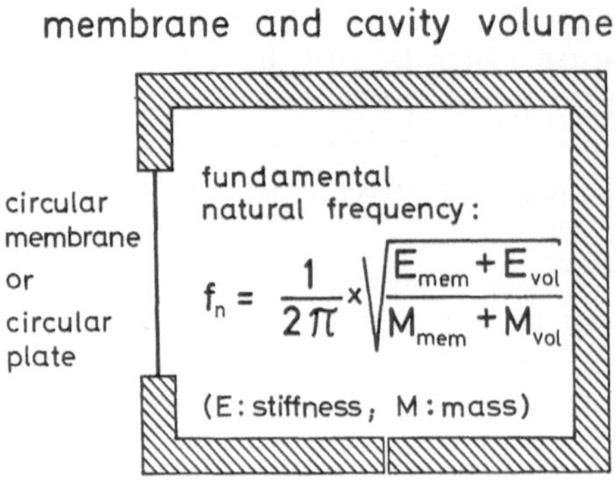

## membrane and cavity volume

fundamental
natural frequency:

circular
membrane
or
circular
plate

$$f_n = \frac{1}{2\pi} \times \sqrt{\frac{E_{mem} + E_{vol}}{M_{mem} + M_{vol}}}$$

(E: stiffness, M: mass)

stiffness of the cavity volume $\quad E_{vol} = \dfrac{c^2 \times \rho \times A^2}{V}$

    c = velocity of sound in air
    $\rho$ = density of air
    A = area of the membrane (or plate)
    V = volume of the cavity

stiffness of the membrane $\quad E_{mem} = 23.7 \times \sigma \times t$

    $\sigma$ = tension of the membrane
    t = thickness of the membrane

stiffness of the plate $\quad E_{plate} = \dfrac{93.3 \times Y \times t^3}{A}$

    Y = Young's modulus of elasticity
    t = thickness of the plate
    A = area of the plate

Fig. 6. Components determining the fundamental natural frequency of a simple cavity-membrane system. The middle ear is basically an approximation of such an arrangement

crophones, it is a capillary. The membrane has a stiffness due to its tension as well as a mass. Because the ossicular chain is attached to the tympanic membrane, it also contributes to both elasticity and mass of the membrane.

Although air is compressible, it offers resilient resistance. That is why the volume of such a cavity essentially acts like a spring. The capillary shown is functionally closed for all but the extremely low frequencies. Taking all this into account we can approximate the natural frequency of the cavity-membrane system in the way shown in Fig. 6. For such a system the fundamental natural frequency is that frequency band to which the apparatus is most sensitive. This frequency rises with increasing stiffness of both membrane and air volume; it decreases with increasing mass of both membrane and air volume. The latter term is the "effective mass of the air volume," only about one-third of the value that can be determined by measuring the cavity volume.

Besides the mass, the other important components are the stiffness of both the cavity volume and the membrane. The formula given shows that the stiffness of the volume increases with the square of the area of the membrane. It also shows that it increases with decreasing volume. In other words: of two ears with the same volume the ear with a larger tympanic membrane has a higher volume stiffness. Also, of two ears with identical membrane areas the ear with a smaller middle ear cavity has a higher stiffness of the cavity volume. Since the volume elasticity increases with the square of the membrane area, it is about proportional to the fourth power of the ear's linear dimension. The elasticity decreases with the volume, hence with about the third power of the linear dimension of the ear. Therefore the stiffness of the cavity volume will increase with the dimension of the ear, unless modified ratios between membrane area and cavity volume compensate for this. This volume-stiffness is defined as force per displacement.

Ignoring for the moment that the ossicles are attached to the tympanic membrane in the mammalian ear, we now consider the membrane and its influence. Figure 6 shows that the stiffness of a membrane depends on its internal tension and its thickness, assuming that both remain constant throughout the membrane. The membrane mass is the product of the area, the thickness, and the density of the material. These four basic elements determine the fundamental natural frequency of such a simple cavity-membrane system: the stiffness of the air volume and of the membrane and the mass of the air volume and the membrane. Variations of these parameters permit the natural frequency of such a system to be set at any desired value with restrictions of course because of material properties.

Since it is easy to make a small membrane reasonably stiff it is no problem to give a high natural frequency to such a small system. Similarly, it is easy to give a low natural frequency to a large system. Nature, however, has to solve many problems simultaneously and sometimes the more common solution cannot be carried out for other reasons. If a large system has to be given a high natural frequency and the cavity volume has to be very large for one reason or another, then the membrane has to be very stiff to compensate for the low stiffness of the cavity volume. Thus, a point may be reached where no membrane can be made stiff enough; this actually happened in some dolphins, as will be shown later. These animals overcame this obstacle by replacing the tympanic membrane by a bony plate, which gave them the stiffness necessary. Figure 6 shows that the stiffness of such a plate depends on Young's modulus of elasticity, its area, but most of all its thickness. Thus, membrane thickness is the parameter that facilitates regulation of stiffness. The mass of the plate is the product of area, thickness, and density. Otherwise the plate is similar to the membrane.

At this point a brief discussion is useful concerning the various opinions on the tension of the tympanic membrane. Helmholtz (1868) assumed that at least the circular fibers of the tympanic membrane are elastic and under tension. In 1949 v. Békésy found that the tympanic membrane in human cadavers is not a stretched membrane but resembles a stiffened cone. In the ventral part of the membrane a fold was assumed to indicate the absence of tension. This is important because Helmholtz (1868) believed the tympanic membrane itself to act as an amplifier of the sound pressure on the membrane through its curvature and tension. Wever and Lawrence (1954) discussed the problem in detail. Their own experiments indicated that the membrane does not act as a lever as supposed by Helmholtz. Later in 1970 Tonndorf and Khanna studied the vibration of the tympanic membrane in the cat with time-averaging holography and concluded that part of the transformer action of the middle ear resides in the tympanic membrane itself as indicated by Helmholtz.

Within the frame work of this concept the lever action of the tympanic membrane will not be treated. This does not mean that it is assumed to be nonexistent. However, its contribution to the middle ear function seems to be minor, and, given the enormous changes due to the variations of other parameters, this effect will be omitted for the sake of simplicity.

Observations by the author in a large number of anesthetized mammals indicate that the tympanic membrane is stretched. A fold such as described by v. Békésy (1949) was not seen. Probing reveals that the membrane is highly elastic, especially in laboratory rats (*Rattus*) and mice (*Mus*), but the membrane appears to be rather stiff in bats. An interesting feature can be seen in the pangolin (*Manis*). In these animals the tympanic bone is hollow and the tympanic membrane is attached to a blood sponge at its perimeter, a situation discovered by Eschweiler (1899). Manipulation shows that blood can easily move within the sponge and also that the membrane is highly elastic in all directions. The tension of the membrane seems without doubt readily altered by the amount of blood within the spongy tissue.

Nearly all mammals have a structure in their ear not mentioned in Fig. 6, the pars flaccida of the tympanic membrane. As its name indicates it has no tension; it is a thin membrane, often with folds and wrinkles. When sound reaches the ear, both tympanic membrane and pars flaccida are pushed inward although to different degrees. The size of such a flaccid membrane will, therefore, influence the volume stiffness, as shown in Fig. 6. With increasing combined area of pars flaccida and tympanic membrane the stiffness of the cavity volume increases. To simplify matters, the term "stiffness of the cavity volume" will mean that corrections for the pars flaccida have already been made, thus indicating the actual stiffness of the real cavity volume of the ear. In Figs. 3 and 7 the pars flaccida can be seen above the malleus, thus closing the dorsal part of the outer acoustic meatus.

From the previous discussion it follows that the animals size is umimportant, as far as the performance of a single ear is concerned. For the directionality of hearing, however, the distance between both ears is important, but this topic will not be dealt with here. Many zoologists have observed that mammals living in deserts or semi-desert areas tend to have enlarged middle ears. Weber (1927) was already familar with this effect and later it was emphasized again by Heim de Balsac (1936), Zavattari (1936), Legouix et al. (1954), Petter (1953), Wisner et al. (1954), Webster (1961, 1962), Fleischer (1973a), and others. Much speculation has ensued as to the underlying reason for this expanded volume of the middle ear cavity. Webster (1962) showed experimentally in the kangaroo rat (*Dipodomys*) that the ear is very sensitive to low frequencies and that replacing part of the air in the middle ear with plasticine made the ear less sensitive.

The discussion on the middle ear in desert mammals has been clouded by a basic misconception. Practically everyone describes the auditory bullae as "enormous" or "extraordinarily voluminous," or the like. These animals however, do not have middle ears that are exceptionally large. All the species with such specialized ears are small. This is what surprises everyone, to find a medium-size ear in a small-size animal. Mammalogists however are concerned about the *relative* size of these ears. The skull of *Microdipodops,* for example, a small desert mouse, presents an amazing sight — half of the head seems to be ear. The question arises as to what small desert mammals gain by increasing the middle ear?

A single ear functions well independent of the size of the head containing it. Yet the sense of hearing is inseparably linked to the biology of the animal. Deserts and semi-deserts are areas with low background noise and are also characterized by open space. Brush and shrubs occur only occasionally without any continuous cover of grass. Thus locomotion is hardly obstructed by such obstacles, suggesting the underlying cause for these small dessert dwellers being all outstanding runners and jumpers.

Usually they are bipedal with highly specialized hind limbs; the Heteromyidae are called kangaroo rats and kangaroo mice because of this. Using another expression, we can say that the *"biologic distance"* is large in these small species. The *"biologic distance"* is that portion of its environment which is, under normal conditions of interest to the animal. Of course, this distance depends on the morphologic structure of the environment and the locomotive abilities of the species. For a shrew in the underbrush the biologic distance may be half a meter or a meter at the most. Anything beyond that is "remote" to the animal. For a lion, on the other hand, the *biologic distance* measures in kilometers and to a high-flying vulture 10 miles may still be within its *biologic distance.*

The question now arises as to how a larger biologic distance, of one or several hundred meters, is related to the size of the ears. The major reason for this is a peculiarity of physical acoustics. Sound intensity from a small sound source, such as an animal, decreases with the square of the distance from the source, a peculiarity independent of the frequency. In addition to this the atmospheric attenuation of sound increases with the frequency. In other words, high frequencies do not travel very far, because they rapidly fade away due to atmospheric attenuation. Low frequencies, on the other hand, undergo only small amounts of atmospheric attenuation and consequently travel farther. This relation is a very fundamental one for the evolution of hearing, especially in connection with the relation between frequency and informational content of sound. The amount of information to be gained from sound waves increases with the frequency. Thus, high frequency sound can carry a lot of information, while low frequency sound is poor in informational content. Since high frequencies are rapidly attenuated with distance, a compromise has to be made. Either a lot of information can be transferred or received over a small distance, or a small amount of information can be transferred or received over a large distance. Such a compromise has to be made in every acoustic system, be it technical or biologic, in the desert or in the ocean. In the latter case the acoustic properties of water have to be included, but otherwise the situation is the same.

The desert mammals, therefore should clearly have ears that are sensitive to those frequencies that can travel at least their biologic distance without being attenuated below audibility. Hence they need low-frequency ears, but this is not easy to achieve if the ears are reasonably small. In order to make the ear sensitive the ear drum is increased in these animals. From Fig. 6 it is obvious that the volume of the cavity has to be increased drastically to reduce the stiffness of the cavity volume, since this would raise the natural frequency. The stiffness of the tympanic membrane should also be reduced to tune the ear to low frequencies. Modifications of the ossicular chain are also necessary, but they will be discussed later.

Moles are a special case, since in their tube system high frequencies are rapidly absorbed by the surface of the walls, while low frequencies can travel rather far. The development of low-frequency ears within this group is, therefore, understandable. The situation of a mole within its tube system is acoustically quite similar to the mechanical arrangement of a spider sitting in its net. This extended network of "acoustic antennas" may be responsible for the well-known emigration of the European mole (*Talpa*) from areas regularly cut by motorized lawn mowers, probably in order to escape the frightening noise.

In summary, the ear has to have a certain volume if it must be sensitive to low frequencies. This happens normally in larger animals and the ear is not remarkable because the head is large. If biologic reasons force small animals to develop low frequency ears the ear seems at first to be surprisingly large relative to the small animal. Finding exactly the same ear in a larger species would not seem remarkable. This connection between the biologic distance of the animal and the size of the ear can also be used to some extent to determine the biology in extinct mammals. Such an approach, however, should be used with caution because other factors not mentioned may also be of importance.

So far the volume of the middle ears considered has been described as filled with air and similar to that shown to the left in Fig. 7. In many mammals, including all the small desert dwellers just discussed this is the case. They have a large cavity volume relative to the tympanic membrane and the form of the cavity is more or less spherical. In many species some ridges or incomplete walls separate the middle ear cavity incompletely into several subspaces. Some of the ridges undoubtedly prevent vibrations of the wall, especially where the bone is extremely thin and light.

In quite a number of mammals however, the middle ear cavity is filled with a bony meshwork not unlike sponges in form. A great many bony spicules together form the three-dimensional meshwork. Inside the meshwork there is air and it is in contact with that of the unobstructed portion of the middle ear cavity. Figure 7 shows two such ears with bony meshwork. All kinds of intermediate stages exist between an ear without and with such cancellous bone. The first step towards a bony meshwork seems to be radial ridges starting from the outer margin of the tympanic membrane. Then a few pillars cross the cavity volume and when their number increases a meshwork is formed. The meshes, large at first, can then gradually decrease in size. To be sure, these changes are evolutionary ones. Each species has a typical degree of meshwork (if one at all) and it remains so throughout the adult life of the animal.

Many mammalogists have described these structures. Kolmer (1913) found it in the European mole (*Talpa*); Herre (1953) described it in the Tylopoda; and Hooper (1968) showed it for a number of Microtine rodents, to mention just a few researchers. The distribution of this meshwork is indeed puzzling. Whereas some small mammals like some voles (*Microtus*) or the ermine (*Mustela*) have it, the rats (*Rattus*), the mice (*Mus* and *Apodemus*), and the bats do not have it. The pigs (*Sus*) and the hippopotamus (*Hippopotamus*) have the meshwork in the ear, as do horses (*Equus*) and cattle (*Bos*), but it is not developed in the giraffe (*Giraffa*). In the elephants (*Loxodonta* and *Elephas*) the beginning of a loose meshwork is present. Obviously the meshwork appears independent of the size of the animal and it cannot be linked to a specific habitat.

In a comparative study Fleischer (1973a) found that such a bony meshwork is correlated to a reduced volume of the cavity, as compared to similar ears without this meshwork. Especially ears with a volume greatly deviating from a spherical configuration have this meshwork. The need to reshape the bulla is not that uncommon. Herre (1953) recognized that in the New World camel, Lama, the auditory bulla id wedged between the lower jaw and the hyoid bone, a situation which prevents the middle ear from being more or less spherical. The skull in the mole (*Talpa*) is so flat that no space is left for a voluminous middle ear cavity; the same holds true for the ermine (*Mustela*). In general the middle ear cavity is relocated to some extent, if there is not sufficient space for a spherical form (see Fig. 7). The necessary air volume is thus stored in interstices of the head. We do not have to look very far to find another example. Since the base of the skull in man is much too crowded to permit true auditory bullae the middle ear cavities extended into the squamosal to secure the volume required.

20

## configuration of some middle ear cavities

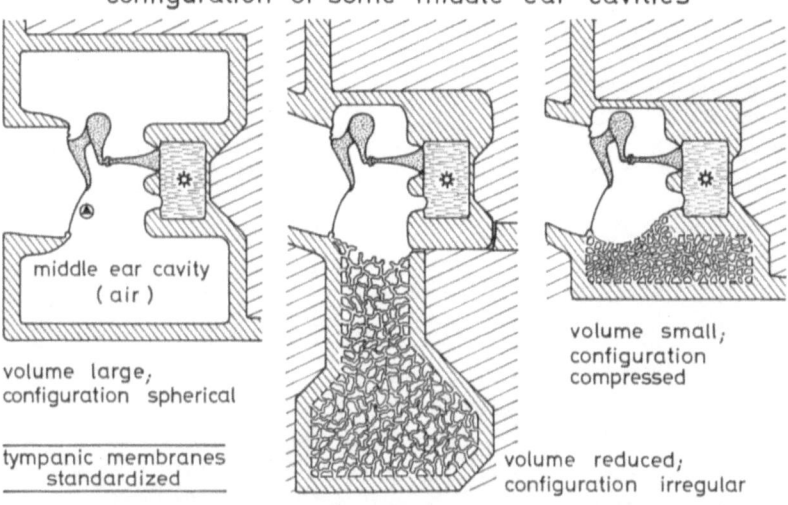

middle ear cavity
(air)

volume large;
configuration spherical

tympanic membranes
standardized

volume small;
configuration
compressed

volume reduced;
configuration irregular

Fig. 7. Appearance of spongy bone inside the middle ear cavity of many mammalian species. It is characteristic for ears with a relatively large tympanic membrane and a cavity deviating considerably from a spherical configuration. In this way resonance is suppressed by increasing turbulence and friction within the middle ear

The relationships in Fig. 6 show that the reduced cavity volume, associated with the cancellous bone in the middle ear, increases the stiffness of the system. This increased stiffness will sharpen the resonance, i. e., the ear becomes very nonlinear in the region of the natural frequency. To suppress this undesirable effect, the internal surface is greatly increased by the introduction of the meshwork. This drastically increases the friction at the surface, as well as the turbulence during vibration, which in turn dampens the system, thus reducing the strong resonance. Such a solution is also applied in some high-quality loudspeakers to suppress unwanted resonances. The extremely rugged surface of the cellulae mastoideae in man is the functional equivalent of the cancellous bone in the bullae of the mammals mentioned. All these structures help to overcome the resonance problems if an ordinary middle ear cavity is not feasible due to lack of adequate space.

## 5. Tympanic Membrane and Tympanic Plate

Since mammals descended from terrestrial forms and the overwhelming majority of them remained terrestrial, it is not surprising that the mammalian ear is a terrestrial one. The middle ear is therefore a device to match the acoustic impedances of air and the liquids in the inner ear. To achieve this a membrane acts as the receiving area for airborne sound. Coupled to this membrane is a mechanical system, the auditory ossicles, which amplifies the pressure in part at the expense of the displacement. The last element is the output area of the middle ear, the footplate of the stapes, which is identical with the input area of the cochlea. A primarily aquatic ear does not need such a middle ear, because the acoustic impedance of sea water is practically identical to that

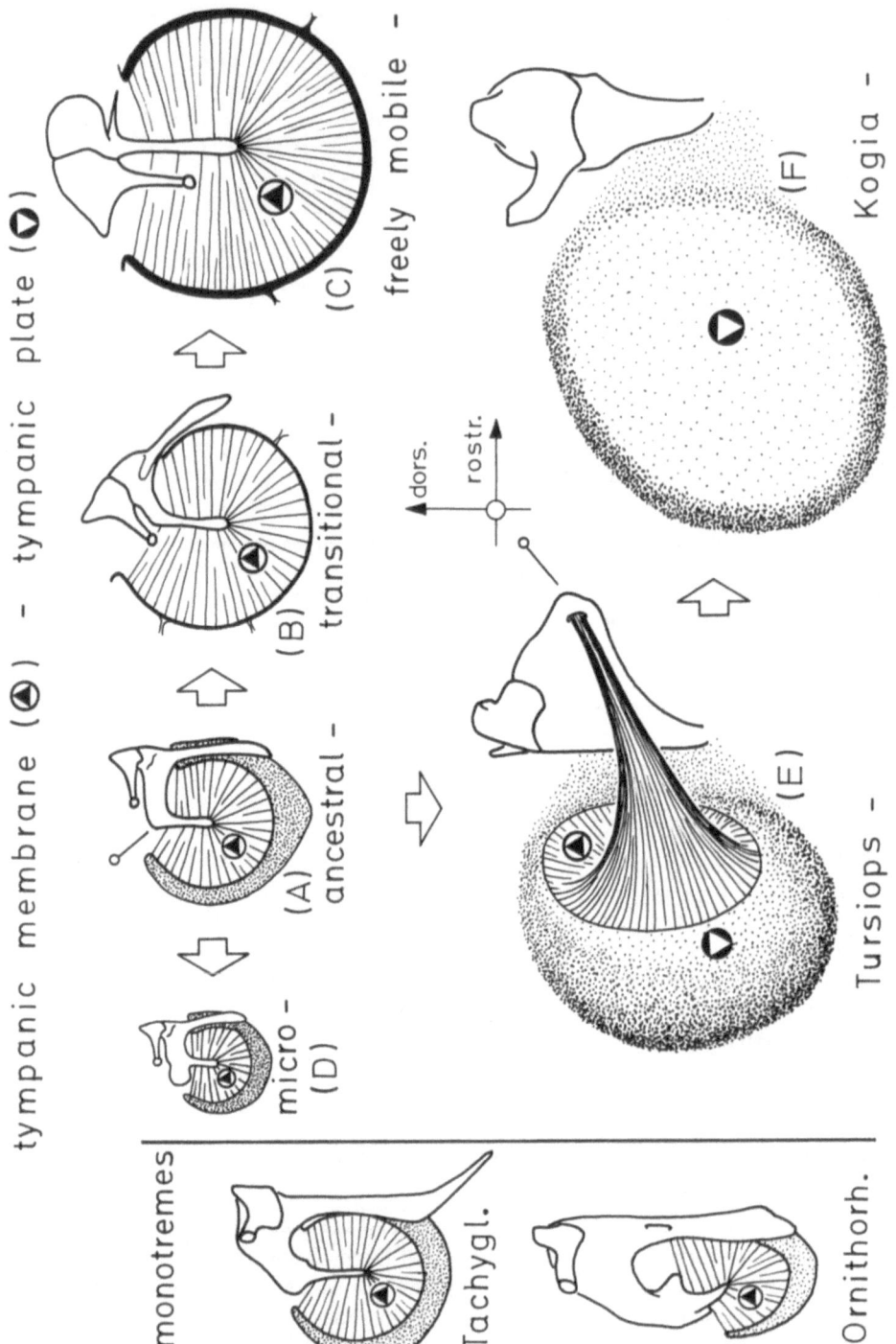

Fig. 8. Evolutionary radiation of the malleus-incus complex and the tympanic membrane, as well as its derivative, as worked out by the author. Seen from the side of the brain. Orientation standardized. The tympanic plate consists of dense, ceramiclike bone. *Tursiops* and *Kogia* are both cetaceans. − *needle* pointing to corresponding parts of the malleus in ancestral and *Tursiops*-type middle ear

of the perilymph and endolymph within the inner ear. Mammals adapted to an aquatic life have to adjust a basically terrestrial ear to the requirements of hearing under water. Despite the fact that considerable morphologic changes are often involved, it is nevertheless always apparent that such aquatic ears are modified terrestrial ones.

Except for a small number of specialized odontocetes, all mammals have tympanic membranes (Fig. 8). Monotremes are no different in this respect from marsupials and placentals. In terrestrial forms, including the seals, the tympanic membrane is somewhat conical, because the tip of the manubrium pulls the membrane somewhat toward the middle ear cavity. Only the pars tensa is shown in the drawing. As the name indicates it appears to be under tension, because no wrinkles or folds appear. Probing the tympanic membrane in anesthetized animals reveals the membrane to be quite elastic. Unfortunately no details as to the stiffness of the tympanic membranes throughout the mammals are available.

Diameter and area of the membrane differ to a great extent among the species. In *Suncus etruscus,* a minute shrew, the membrane diameter is only 1.2 mm, while the African elephant, *Loxodonata africana,* has a membrane diameter of 31 - 33 mm. Thus the membrane areas are 1.13 mm$^2$ and $\sim$ 800 mm$^2$, respectively, i. e., in terrestrial forms the membrane areas vary within a range of 1 - over 700. Although it is true that small species in general have small tympanic membranes, the area of the membrane is not a function of the size or weight of the animal, but depends on the hearing capability. That is why the little chinchilla has a larger membrane than, say, the giraffe. As mentioned earlier, the small desert dwellers also have membranes larger than those in other mammals of comparable body size. More measurements can be found in Fleischer (1973a).

The shape of the tympanic membrane is not uniform, but varies between a somewhat curved u, as in many carnivores and ungulates, and a nearly perfect circle. The latter form is common in those ears where the middle ear cavity is voluminous and spherical in configuration. Experiments on the functional significance of these differences have not been conducted, but this factor does not seem to be of great importance for hearing.

Before dealing with the ear in aquatic mammals, some properties of sound will be mentioned. First of all sound travels $\sim$ 4.5-times faster under water than in air. But more importantly, for the same sound intensity the pressure is about 62 times greater in water than it is in air. Since the mammalian ear is basically a pressure receiver, this translates into a 62-fold increase in the force available to drive the middle ear, if the area of the tympanic membrane remains constant. Displacement of the water particles is 62-times less than it is for air particles at the same intensity and frequency. Thus the favorable pressure relation facilitates the ear's reception of sound under water.

The tympanic membrane in the Pinnipedia is much tougher than in terrestrial forms, but otherwise no significant specializations seem to be present. The auditory ossicles, however, are usually much heavier in these animals than in terrestrial forms of similar cochlear size. A unique peculiarity is found among the Sirenia. The tympanic membrane in these mammals is also tough, but, contrary to the condition found in other mammals, it is bulged outward by the sturdy manubrium of the malleus. Sirenias have large tympanic membranes with a diameter of $\sim$ 20 mm. Their auditory ossicles (Fig. 17) are very heavy and massive, possibly one of the reasons for the large tympanic membrane. More details can be found in Robineau (1969) and Fleischer (1971).

Cetaceans have a highly modified hearing organ, so much so that the components often cannot be easily recognized. One of the fundamental changes is a rotation of the entire malleus-incus complex (Fleischer, 1973c). This evolutionary rotation is common to all cetaceans and must have occurred early in their evolution. During this evolutionary rotation part of the tympanic membrane was stretched into a conical ligament, which is attached to the malleus (see Fig. 8). As shown by Fleischer (1973a) the malleus in cetaceans has no manubrium. Instead the tympanic ligament, as this conical extension of the tympanic membrane is called, is attached to the transversal part of the malleus in the *Tursiops*-type ear. In Fig. 8 the *tip of the needle* points to corresponding parts pf the malleus in the ancestral type and the *Tursiops*-type middle ear. Another view of tympanic membrane, tympanic ligament, and ossicular chain is presented in Fig. 16. Many odontocetes and all mysticetes have the *Tursiops*-type of tympanic membrane.

A condition as unusual as this needs some explanation. As mentioned earlier a membrane is ineffective at high frequencies, i. e., above its fundamental natural frequency, because it then vibrates in segments and no longer as a unit. Another problem at higher frequencies ist that the force applied to the manubrium acts predominantly perpendicular to the surface of the membrane. If the membrane extends into a ligament, as it does in the *Tursiops*-type, the force applied to the malleus acts along the direction of the tympanic ligament, a situation highly favorable at high frequencies. Since it is futile to push a string or a ligament, it is necessary to keep the entire system — malleus, tympanic ligament, and tympanic membrane — under tension. The resilience is supplied by the malleus, which is fused to the tympanic bone (see Sect. 6). In this way the tympanic membrane is also supplied with tension. The tympanic membrane in dolphins is exceptionally strong. Fleischer (1973b) found that the tympanic ligament in *Tursiops* is able to lift weights of up to 1.95 kg. Such great strength can only be developed through adaptation to dynamic forces, because both ends of the tympanic ligaments are attached to structures that are nowhere nearly as strong as to require such tensile strength.

As regards the area of the tympanic membrane, the cetaceans can clearly be divided into two distinct groups. Dolphins have relatively small membranes, while the mysticetes have large ones. The tympanic membrane in *Tursiops* measures 7mm by 10 mm, in *Stenella* it is slightly smaller, and in *Pseudorca* it is somewhat larger, measuring 7 mm by 11 mm. Mysticetes have the largest membranes among living mammals. A specimen of *Eubalaena glacialis* had a membrane of 30 mm by 40 mm, and a membrane of 35 mm by 37 mm was found in *Eubalaena sieboldii.* Even the small minke whale (*Balaenoptera acutorostrata*) has a tympanic membrane of 25 mm by 30 mm. (For the sake of completeness it has to be mentioned that in the mysticetes the pars flaccida protrudes into the outer acoustic meatus, forming a blind sac.)

More is involved in the cetacean ear than just the specialized tympanic membrane. Figure 5 shows the tympanic bone with its opening for the tympanic membrane. To be sure, in reality the circumference of the tympanic membrane is surrounded by several flanges and processes of the tympanic bone, so that the membrane is barely visible from the outside, if at all. Hence, Fig. 5 shows the basic relation, omitting some structural details. Nevertheless, the bone surrounding the membrane is seen to be thin. The pictograph used for this thin bone is also shown in the *Tursiops*-type ear in Fig. 8 as well as in Fig. 16. Especially the latter drawing clearly demonstrates that both the membrane and the thin portion of the tympanic bone form the interface between the soft body tissues (predominantly fat) and the air of the middle ear cavity. Such a thin bone will certainly vibrate and its vibration will be transmitted to the malleus via the tympanic ligament.

From the theoretical aspect the thin bony portion must be included in the receiving area for sound. In other words, the receiving area is composed of two major components, a membrane and an area of thin bone adjacent to the membrane. The various species show great differences in the size of this bony portion. In Fig. 8 the thin bone is lightly *stippled*. Its thickness gradually increases with the distance from the tympanic membrane. Of course this is a simplification for the purpose of illustrating the principle, but detailed measurements of this thin portion have been made by Fleischer (1973c, 1975). Dolphins have an irregularly shaped portion, but always next to the membrane. The thick medial rim shown in Fig. 5 surrounds the thin bony part both medially and occipitally, thus forming a frame for the thin portion, stable at higher frequencies because of its inertia.

In the mysticetes the thin portion is only rudimentally developed. In fact, only someone who is familiar with this structure in the dolphins and thus knows what to look for can find it. In summary many odontocetes, as well as the mysticetes, have the morphologic type, *Tursiops*-type, middle ear.

During his studies of the dolphin middle ear Fleischer (1975) came across the ear of *Kogia,* the pygmy sperm whale, which does not have a tympanic membrane. This was a surprise, because it was not only the first known mammal without a tympanic membrane, it is also an animal that uses a sonar system based upon ultrasonic sound. An analysis of the situation revealed that in this species the thin bony portion of the tympanic bone has replaced the entire tympanic membrane (Fig. 8). Since this bony plate replaced the tympanic membrane it was called *"tympanic plate."* It consists of dense, ceramiclike bone and has a thickness of 1/3 - 3/5 mm. Its dimensions are ∿ 7 mm by 12 mm, but with an irregular shape. *Kogia* is no unique exception among cetaceans. At least *Physeter,* the sperm whale, has also been proven to lack a tympanic membrane and evidence suggests that this may also hold true for *Berardius, Ziphius,* and *Mesoplodon.* Hence the cetaceans can be divided into two groups, one with a tympanic membrane and the other without a membrane but with the tympanic plate. This is without doubt an extremely specialized type of middle ear which has evolved from a *Tursiops*-type ear.

Discussion in the preceding chapter clearly indicates that such a bony plate increases the stiffness of the sound-receiving area, which in turn favors the reception of high frequencies. Dolphins generally have high-tuned middle ears and the tympanic membrane, or tympanic plate, is only one element. Although they should have problems with the lower frequencies, this is not the case because of the mechanism discussed in connection with Fig. 5.

Diving is a special problem for the hearing organ, because the pressure increases with depth. As far as ordinary soft tissues are concerned this is not important, because physically they are practically noncompressible as is water. (Caisson disease is irrelevant from the aspect of hearing.) However air is easily compressible, so that the tympanic membrane bulges more and more into the middle ear cavity during diving. If no countermeasures are taken the tympanic membrane ruptures at a certain depth, a catastrophic situation for an aquatic mammal depending on its sense of hearing.

The volume of an air-filled cavity under water can be derived from the law of Boyle-Mariotte, which states that the product of the pressure (P) and the volume (V)

## adaptations for deep diving

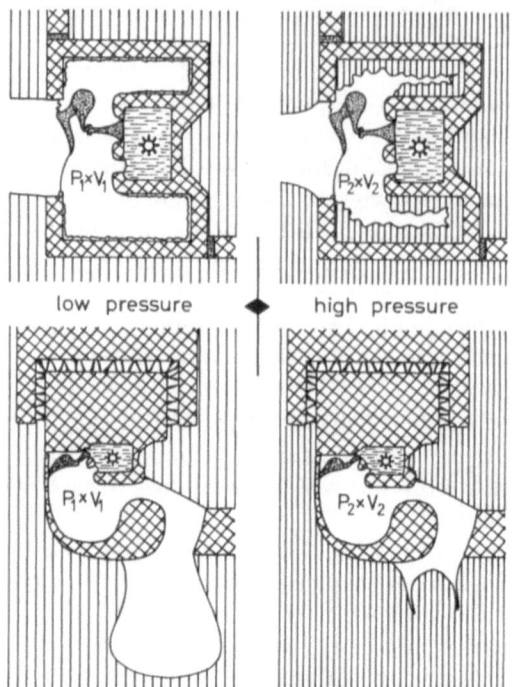

low pressure          high pressure

Fig. 9. During deep diving the pressure inside and outside the middle ear has to be kept about equal. This can be done by filling cavernous tissue inside the cavity with blood (*above*) or by decreasing the volume of accessory air spaces (*below*) $P_1 \times V_1 \sim P_2 \times V_2$

remains constant (air is treated as an ideal gas and at constant temperature.) Thus, if the pressure during diving doubles, the volume of the air will be half the previous value in order to have the same pressure as the surrounding soft tissues. If the volume of the middle ear cavity is somehow reduced, corresponding to the increased pressure, the tympanic membrane will neither be bulged inward nor outward. Of course, rupturing will then be avoided.

The middle ear cavity should thus not be constant, but rather decrease in volume as the pressure increases during diving. The two basic principles for achieving this are shown in the schematic drawing of Fig. 9. The middle ear in seals is a reasonably closed box (*top*), but it is covered inside with a layer of cavernous tissue. As the animals dive, blood is forced into it, thus reducing the volume of the cavity. Morphologic details can be found in Møhl (1968) and Repenning (1972), among others.

Many dolphins also have such a cavernous tissue, but it is more or less like a rag, lying inside the tympanic cavity. As of now no principal difference between both forms has been ascertained. In both cases blood is forced into the cavernous tissue during diving, thus reducing the volume of the cavity.

Another way of achieving the same goal is to reduce the volume of accessory air sacs outside the middle ear, as long as it is part of the same volume (*bottom* of Fig. 9). A special way is to reduce the volume of the lungs during diving and connect the middle ear volume via the Eustachian tube to it. This is the way human divers achieve equalization of the pressure inside and outside the middle ear. Hence the lungs can be considered the equivalent of an external extension of the middle ear cavity, so that it is a special case of the situation shown in the *lower part* of Fig. 9. Needless to say, all mechanisms mentioned can function at once.

Of importance is the depth to which the animal is capable of diving safely. Sirenia do not need special adaptation for diving. Since the aquatic plants they feed on all grow near the surface for adequate sunlight, these animals have no need to dive to great depths. However, their middle ear cavity is not surrounded by bone ventrally (Fig. 4), so that it can decrease in volume during diving. The situation is different in many, if not all, marine cetaceans because they may dive several hundred meters. Unfortunately no exact data on the diving habits seem to be available, except for the sperm whale (*Physeter*), which feeds on the large cephalopods of the ocean bottom. During these ventures into the lightless depth they occasionally get entangled in deep-sea cables and strangle to death (Heezen, 1957). These heavy cables lie on the floor of the ocean and are chewed up by the struggling sperm whales. Repair crews have found many choked specimens of *Physeter,* and thereby established that these animals dive at least to 1135 meters. The mechanisms for pressure equalization are not known in detail, but it can be assumed that both basic principles are operative to achieve this feat. An interesting sidelight can be derived from Fig. 6. During deep diving the frequency response of the ear changes, predominantly because of the increased stiffness of the air volume in the middle ear cavity.

The inner ear is a liquid-filled system and as such insensitive to changes in pressure. Hence no cochlear specializations are known which are exclusively due to the aquatic environment of the animal. Experiments with guinea pigs by McNall and Chambers (1972) seem to support the assumption that the cochlea is not sensitive to pressure changes.

# 6. Malleus-Incus Complex

Except for the cyclostomes (hagfishes and lampreys), all vertebrates have jaws. Upper and lower jaw are connected via the quadrate bone and the articular bone, a condition common to all groups but the mammals. This primary articulation is replaced in mammals by the secondary articulation, which is formed by the squamosal and the dentary. The primary articulation, along with two other bony elements, is incorporated into the mammalian otic region: the quadrate (= incus), the articular (= malleus), the gonial (= proc. Folianus of the malleus), and the angular (= tympanic). These relations were discovered long ago and are now universally accepted as the theory of Reichert and Gaupp. Much speculation has focused on the underlying reason for these fundamental evolutionary changes in the mammalian otic region.

From the aspect of the auditory organ, two different events can be separated, although both no doubt occurred simultaneously. The first is the attachment of the tympanic bone to the otic region. This bony element permitted the specialized middle ear cavities to develop, because it is a new element for the ear which can be specially modified to accomodate the needs of the auditory organ. The second event is the expansion of the sound-transmitting apparatus. Previously, in the reptiles, only the columella (= stapes) was present, but in mammals malleus and incus were added to form the ossicular chain. The gonial serves only to anchor the malleus at the tympanic bone (see Fig. 1). To simplify matters, the three components, incus plus malleus and gonial together, will be termed the malleus-incus complex.

Before dealing with the details of the auditory organ, an interesting similarity between the primary articulation of the vertebrate jaw and the malleus-incus complex will be treated. The quadrate in nonmammals forms the convex, and the articular, the concave part of the articulation. This basic relation is maintained throughout the extensive evolutionary radiation of the mammalian malleus-incus complex, i. e., the incus forms the convex, and the malleus, the concave part of the malleus-incus articulation (see Figs. 1, 8 and 15). Monotremes, however, prove the exception.

At this point ist seems appropriate to justify the treatment of the malleus-incus complex as a functional unit. One reason is that in quite a number of mammals malleus and incus are fused, so that both function without doubt as a unit. Since this happens in some forms with a great sensitivity of hearing, e. g., the chinchilla, it cannot be considered degenerative. In general, malleus and incus seem to function together, as will be discussed more thoroughly later. Another reason is the addition of this complex to the stapes during the early evolution. But more important is the unit's semi-independence from the stapes. In other words, the long arm of the incus is connected to the stapes via an intercalated soft lamella of cartilage, without any known exceptions. Because of this elastic element in between, the ossicular chain is functionally composed of two elements: the malleus-incus complex and the stapes.

The evolutionary radiation of the malleus-incus complex was analyzed by Fleischer (1973a). In this study the size of the various hearing organs was measured and indicated, yet in the summary of the evolutionary changes the ossicles were standardized in size. Further studies, especially dealing with the cetaceans as well as with some desert-living mammals, made it perfectly clear that the size of the ear is of critical importance. A simplified summary of the radiation of the mammalian malleus-incus complex, based upon the author's analyses, is presented in Fig. 10. The monotremes are omitted, because their ear is principally different, as far as the complex is concerned and, moreover, they may not be true mammals. Needless to say, the evolutionary changes are continuous and the types indicated only serve to simplify the discussion.

Apparently the size of the ear is related to the configuration of the malleus-incus complex. However, the relation is not a rigid one, but rather a strong tendency. Especially the freely mobile type (*C*) occurs in terrestrial forms with medium-size or large tympanic membranes. The microtype (*D*) occurs only in forms with small ears, and, furthermore, all the minute ears show this type, more or less pronounced.

The ancestral type (*A*) has already been discussed in connection with Fig. 1. As its name indicates, this primitive form gave rise to the three major branches of the evolutionary radiation, but it still exists in many mammalian species. It is typically small the diameter of the tympanic membrane is ∿ 3 - 6 mm. The gonial (see Fig. 1) is usually solidly fused with the tympanic bone. Hence the malleus is firmly anchored at the tympanic bone. Such a fusion between both elements, occasionaly caused some bewilderment, although it is quite normal for most mammals. Opposite to the gonial, the short arm of the incus is connected to the periotic bone by means of a short and stubby ligament. Both ossicles are connected via a joint that includes a thin layer of cartilage so that both elements can be separated.

One line of evolutionary adaptation leads to the freely mobile type (*A - B - C*) found in man, the chinchilla, the porcupine (*Hystrix*), the pangolin (*Manis*), and many others. In type (*C*) the gonial is reduced to the anterior process of the malleus

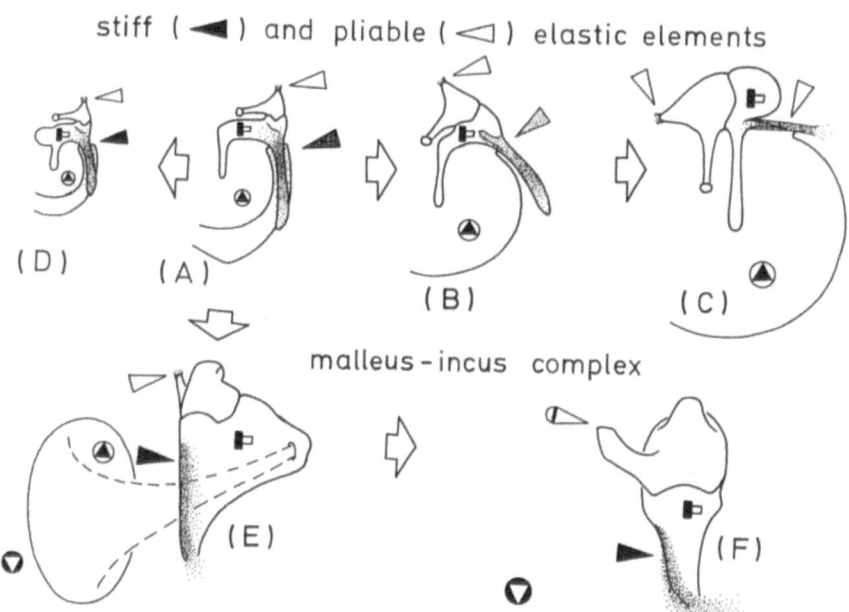

stiff ( ◀ ) and pliable ( ◁ ) elastic elements

(D)  (A)  (B)  (C)

malleus – incus complex

(E)  (F)

Fig. 10. Illustration of the structural elements representing the torsional stiffness ($K$) of the malleus-incus complex, the functional significance of which is outlined in Fig. 11. The malleus-incus complex is anchored at both ends: on one side the gonial is attached to the tympanic bone, while on the other the short arm of the incus is attached to the periotic bone. Elastic elements are *stippled* and their torsional stiffness is indicated by the *darkness of the arrows*. The *capital letters* refer to the types shown in Fig. 8

and the latter is fixed by means of the anterior ligament surrounding the anterior process. Because of this ligamentous connection, the malleus is much less firmly anchored than in type ($A$). The short arm of the incus is again fixed by a short ligament. Besides these two ligaments are normally some folds of soft tissue, such as the superior ligament of malleus and incus in man, but these folds mainly serve nutritional purposes and because they are pliable can be omitted here. The name, freely mobile type, refers to the fact that the malleus and hence the entire malleus-incus complex is no longer fused with the tympanic but only anchored by means of a ligament. In a number of such ears malleus and incus are fused together; rodents seem especially prone to this.

Between the types ($A$) and ($C$) is a transitional type ($B$). Its gonial is less developed than in ($A$), but normally is still fused with the tympanic. In some cases it may be tied to the tympanic by connective tissue. In these forms the anterior ligament begins to appear around the gonial. As shown in Fig. 10, the malleus is more firmly anchored than in ($C$), but less so than in type ($A$). The short arm of the incus is connected to the periotic via a ligament.

A special form of the transitional type is found in the manatees (Sirenia). Unlike the condition found in other mammals, the malleus-incus complex in sirenians is fused with other structures at both ends (Fig. 17). The malleus is fused with the tympanic and the short arm of the incus is fused with the periotic. This peculiarity is found in all modern-day sirenians and was also developed in the now extinct Steller's sea cow (*Hy-*

*drodamalis*). These two fusions notwithstanding, a clear articulation exists between both ossicles, so that malleus and incus are not fused together.

Returning to Fig. 10, we see that another specialization of the ancestral type led to the microtype. The microtypes range in size from 1.2 to ~ 4 mm in diameter of the tympanic membrane. Tympanic and gonial are solidly fused, so that the malleus is anchored rather rigidly. At the end of the short arm of the incus is a short ligament, (*D*). The articulation between malleus and incus is well developed, as in the ancestral and the transitional type. Such a microtype is found in bats (Microchiroptera), shrews (Soricidae), as well as in many rodents such as the common mouse (*Mus*).

In those cetaceans with a tympanic membrane (*Tursiops*-type; E) the malleus is solidly fused with the tympanic, while the short arm of the incus is fixed by a ligament. Malleus and incus are not fused, but separated by an elaborate articulation composed of two unlike facets (see Fig. 15). The baleen whales (Mysticeti) have a longer gonial, so that the transversal part of the malleus appears to be sitting on a short stem. Otherwise the malleus-incus is very similar to the one in *Tursiops* and other dolphins.

As previously mentioned, some of the odontocete cetaceans have lost the tympanic membrane and replaced it by a rigid bony plate, the tympanic plate. Therefore it is no great surprise that their malleus-incus complex is also different from dolphins with a membrane. In the *Kogia*-type (Fig. 10, F) the complex is lighter, but the malleus is also fused with the tympanic (see also Figs. 4 and 5). It is the most reduced malleus among mammals: manubrium as well as transversal part is lost, only the part surrounding the articulation is developed. The phylogenetic rotation of the malleus-incus complex, characteristic for the cetaceans, is also present, revealing that this type derived from an ear of the *Tursiops*-type. Contrary to the situation in other cetaceans, the short arm of the incus is strong and uniquely curved. It is not held by a ligament, but rather has a flat, oval area of contact with the periotic. This contact appears very similar to the contact between incus and stapes. The differences between the anchoring of the incus in both types of cetaceans is shown in Fig. 15 and details will be discussed later.

The malleus-incus complex in man has long been described as a rotational system, with the rotational axis running through the two ligaments indicated in Fig. 10, *C*. Helmholtz (1868) discussed this opinion, which was offered by anatomists before him. It is easy to see such a freely mobile type, because no fusions interfere with the rotations. Looking at the other types of ears, we see that in those cases the malleus is fused with the tympanic, but a rotation of the complex might still be possible, because the short arm of the incus is also anchored, so that both connections might form a rotational axis just as they do in man. Before continuing with the morphologic details, the principles of torsional vibrations will be summarized using Fig. 11.

In the most simple case (*left side*) a slab is held by a rod or bar, which in turn is anchored at an immobile reference mass on either end. The rod runs through the center of mass of the slab, the mass of the rod being negligible. Under these conditions two parameters determine the natural frequency of such a torsional system: one is the torsional constant of the rod (*K*) and the other, the moment of inertia (*I*). The torsional constant indicates the stiffness of the rod; the higher the stiffness, the greater the value of (*K*). The moment of inertia depends on the mass and the distribution of the slab's mass. It is large if the mass is great and much of it is far away from the rotational axis, which runs through the rod. Likewise, it is small if the mass is small and/or centered closely around the axis. The moment of inertia (*I*) can be determined experimentally or it can be computed if the configuration of the oscillating body is known.

# principles of torsional vibrations

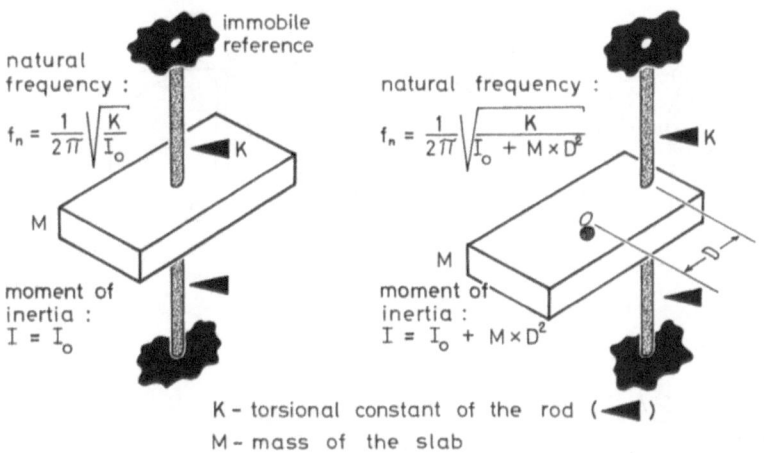

natural frequency :

$$f_n = \frac{1}{2\pi}\sqrt{\frac{K}{I_0}}$$

immobile reference

M

moment of inertia :
$$I = I_0$$

natural frequency :

$$f_n = \frac{1}{2\pi}\sqrt{\frac{K}{I_0 + M \times D^2}}$$

M

moment of inertia :
$$I = I_0 + M \times D^2$$

K – torsional constant of the rod ( ◀ )

M – mass of the slab

axis through center of mass ◆ axis outside center of mass

Fig. 11. Illustration of the Steiner'scher Satz (parallel-axis theorem) and its influence on the natural frequency. The latter can be influenced by variations in the torsional stiffness of the anchoring, but most effectively by shifting the center of mass relative to the rotational axis. Structures representing the torsional stiffness $(K)$ are shown in Fig. 10, while the distribution of mass, relative to the torsional axis $(I_0 + M \times D^2)$ is shown in Fig. 12

In the relation shown in Fig. 11 the natural frequency increases with rising stiffness of the rod and decreases with increasing moment of inertia. A situation in which all the elements are symmetrical, relative to the rotational axis is, however, rare. More likely is a condition in which the rotational axis does not run through the center of mass. If the axis of rotation is shifted from the center of mass but remains parallel to its previous direction, the moment of inertia increases from $I_0$ to $(I_0 + M \times D^2)$. $M$ is the mass of the slab and $D$ is the distance of the center of mass from the new rotational axis. In other words, the moment of inertia increases with the square of the distance between center of mass and rotational axis. This relation is called the Steiner'scher Satz in the German literature and the parallel-axis theorem in the American literature. The natural frequency of such an unbalanced system (on the *right* of Fig. 11) decreases with increasing moment of inertia and $D^2$ is the most influential of the parameters. Hence it is an extremely effective way to tune such a system by altering the distribution of the mass and thus varying the distance between the center of mass and the rotational axis.

Returning to Fig. 10, we see that the torsional stiffness of the rotational axis $(K)$ usually is high at the side of the gonial (*dark arrows*) and weak on the side of the short arm of the incus (*white arrows*). This, however, is no problem, because the two stiffnesses combine to the total rotational stiffness of the malleus-incus complex; thus, the torsional stiffness obviously varies between the types. It is high in cetaceans and in the ancestral and the microtype (*E, F, A* and *D*). The torsional stiffness decreases toward the freely mobile type and is obviously smallest in those forms in which the rotational axis is entirely formed by ligaments, as shown in (*C*).

Even more intriguing is the biologic engineering of the moment of inertia of the malleus-incus complex. This is achieved by altering to a great extent the distribution

31

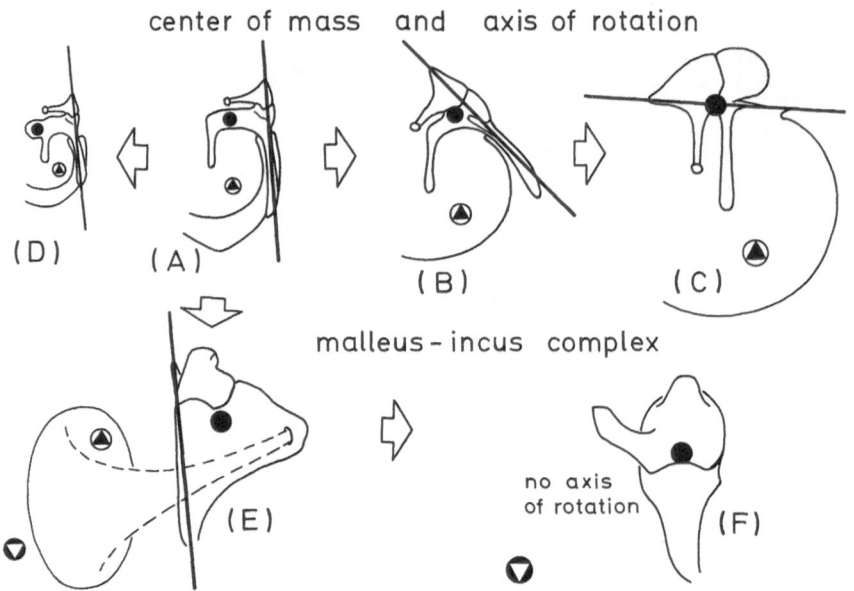

center of mass   and   axis of rotation

(D)  (A)  (B)  (C)

malleus – incus  complex

(E)  no axis of rotation  (F)

Fig. 12. Radiation of the malleus-incus complex with special emphasis on the center of mass and the axis of rotation. In the *Kogia*-type (*F*) no morphologic axis of rotation can be determined. The drawing illustrates the term $(I_o + M \times D^2)$, as defined in Fig. 11. The capital letters refer to the types shown in Figs. 8 and 10

of the mass (Fig. 12). In this way the crucial term $(M \times D^2)$ is varied to achieve the desired moment of inertia. The morphologically determined rotational axis is also delineated.

Preceding the real mammalian ear was the ancestral type (*A*), which was unbalanced because its center of mass was outside the rotational axis somewhere at the transversal part. Of interest is the fact that the incus was relatively small, compared to the malleus. In that line of evolutionary adaptation which led to the freely mobile type (*A - B - C*), drastic changes occurred. The gonial became weaker and weaker, until it was finally replaced by the anterior ligament. The transversal part of the malleus (see Fig. 1) also decreased in size, until the manubrium finally attached to the area of the articulation. A drastic increase of the incus, relative to the malleus, can be observed. Because of this, the incus in the freely mobile type is often as heavy as the malleus and sometimes even more massive. While in the ancestral type (*A*) the rotational axis is almost prallel to the manubrium of the malleus, it changes its direction in such a way that it is almost perpendicular to the manubrium in the freely mobile type. (In a few species such as the mole (*Talpa*) and the elephant (*Loxodonta*) the tilt of the axis has been hindered to some extent by other structures, so that it is not complete.) The part of the articulation in the ancestral type is very small, but it increases in this line of evolution until it is a voluminous structure, called the "head" of the malleus in the human ear. It is clear that such a "head" is a specialized structure and no fundamental component. In some rodents, such as the chinchilla, the head of the malleus and the main body of the incus are elongated and thus rather cylindrical, with the cylinder-axis parallel to the rotational axis.

32

## influence of the orbicular apophysis

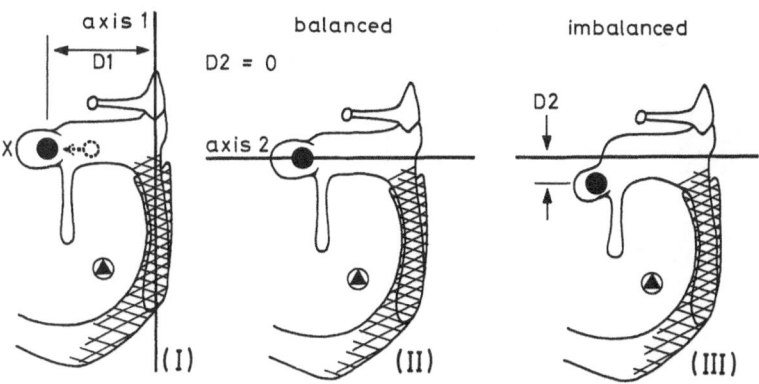

Fig. 13. Malleus-incus complex of the microtype, which is characterized by the orbicular apophysis (*X*), a bulky mass at the base of the manubrium. Mainly because of the apophysis, two major rotational axes are present and the location of the apophysis is of importance relative to both axes

All these changes combined cause the center of mass of the malleus-incus complex to shift ever closer to the roational axis until it is very close to it; some ears may be perfectly balanced, thus reducing the term ($M \times D^2$) to zero. The moment of inertia is then very small, but the torsional stiffness ($K$) is also small because the complex is held by the two ligaments. No exact figures on both parameters are available, but this form of the complex is characteristic for low-frequency ears, such as mans or the chinchillas (mysticetes are different). Such a balanced ear has the advantage that it is insensitive to mechanical shocks because no rotational components exist if the center of mass lies in the axis.

Another specialization is the development of the microtype (Fig. 12, *D*). It is characterized by the orbicular apophysis, which was found and described in rodents by Cockerell et al. (1914). The orbicular apophysis is a bulky mass of bone at the base of the manubrium. It is found in bats (Microchiroptera), many Insectivora, such as the shrews (Soricidae), and in many rodents. In some species it is only a slight bulge or a little hook, while it is enormous in some of the minute shrews. As much as five-sixth of the mass of the malleus can be concentrated in the apophysis. Of course, this additional mass will shift the center of mass of the malleus-incus complex further away from the axis, even beyond the manubrium. Thus starting from the ancestral type, two radically different lines of evolutionary adaptation evidently occurred: in one, the center of mass is shifted toward and finally into the rotational axis, resulting in the freely mobile type. In the other, the center of mass is shifted further away from the axis by the development of the orbicular apophysis, resulting in the microtype. That the microtype is a highly functional ear is easily apparent because it is found in bats, which have a sophisticated sonar system.

However, such an orbicular apophysis complicates matters considerably, especially if it is voluminous, so that it deserves some special attention. The apophysis (*X* in Fig. 13, *I*) increases the distance between the center of mass and the rotational axis, which increases the moment of inertia. Because the torsional stiffness of the axis ($K$) is high, the result is a very high natural frequency, but it will be lowered by the influence of this apophysis (see Fig. 11). At first this may appear puzzling, because the bats have a so-

33

vibrational modes of the
microtype

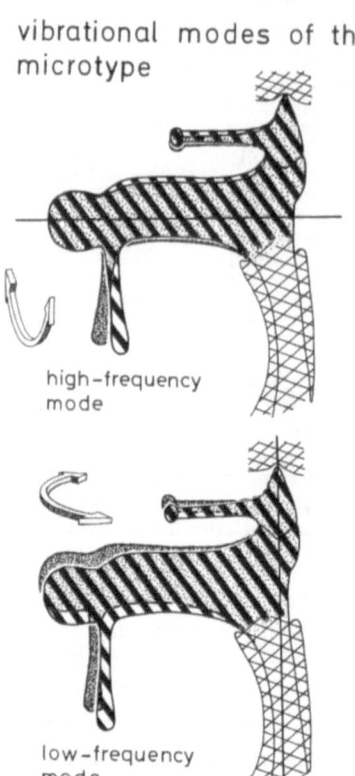

high-frequency
mode

low-frequency
mode

Fig. 14. Illustration of the two major vibratory modes of the microtype, along with the respective rotational axis based on modeling experiments of the author. On the right side the malleus-incus complex is anchored elastically (*cross-hatched areas;* see also Fig. 10). In each vibratory mode two situations 180° out of phase are shown and optically distinguished by *stippling* and *hatching.* The two axes are the same as in Fig. 13

nar system based on high ultrasonic sound. But these animals also have great problems perceiving low frequencies since their middle ear is tuned to extremely high frequencies. Predominantly, this is the result of the minute size and the rigid fusion between the gonial and the tympanic. Without the orbicular apophysis, the natural frequency of the malleus-incus complex might simply be too high, even for the bats. These relations hold true for the other mammals with a microtype ear as well, because the middle ear in bats does not really differ from theirs.

The transversal part in the microtype is normally comparatively thin. Quite often both margins are reinforced so that it resembles an I-beam. Due to this the transversal part can be twisted. The heavy orbicular apophysis will then cause the appearance of another axis of rotation perpendicular to the one discussed. This second axis (Fig. 13, *II, III*) runs along the transversal part of the malleus. The torsional stiffness of the latter results in another, different value of ($K$); the relations shown in Fig. 11 are now valid for the new rotational axis. A survey of the various forms with a microtype reveals that the malleus differs to some extent in configuration. Particularly the orbicular apophysis is not always exactly in the same location, but rather differences occur (see parts *II* and *III* of Fig. 13). If the center of mass is situated outside the second axis it will, of course, lower the natural frequency around that axis.

34

Apparently the orbicular apophysis regulates the natural frequency of the malleus-incus complex around two axes of vibration. Hence, one and the same structure can be used to tune independently the complex in two different vibrational modes, by properly adjusting its position relative to the two vibrational axes. These, to be sure, are theoretical conclusions, because the vibrational modes of the malleus in the microtype have not been studied in nature, only in an enlarged model (Fleischer, 1974). An estimation of the parameters shows that the vibrational mode around *axis 1* is the low-frequency mode (Fig. 14), while the rotation around *axis 2* is the high-frequency mode. So far no experimental data exist on the frequency range of these two vibrational modes. Theoretically it is possible that only one mode is used for hearing, while the other would then be either too high in frequency or too low. Without being able to corroborate it by further evidence, the author assumes that the low-frequency mode is necessary for hearing in the microtype. One reason for this assumption is that in this way nature would keep its old rotational axis (see Fig. 12), which would have simplified the evolutionary adaptations. Whether the high-frequency mode (its natural frequency) is still within the hearing range or above it remains to be determined.

In the high-frequency mode (see Fig. 14) something must yield during the vibrations, considering the fact that the short arm of the incus is tied to the periotic. This may be one reason why the articulation between malleus and incus is so excellently developed, notwithstanding the solid fusion between the gonial and the tympanic bone.

Aside from the tiny species with the microtype, nature also developed giants, at least among the cetaceans. As mentioned earlier, the malleus-incus complex in the *Tursiops*-type is characterized by the evolutionary rotation and in the process by the stretching of part of the tympanic membrane into the tympanic ligament. The transversal part (between the attachment of the tympanic ligament and the articulation) serves as lever for the action of that very ligament. Because the transversal part is rather bulky and cylindrical in cross section, (see Fig. 15) much of the mass of the malleus is concentrated there, the center of mass being located somewhere outside the rotational axis (Fig. 12). Such a strong transversal part seems necessary to prevent buckling at high frequencies, especially in dolphins.

From the evolutionary aspect it is of interest to realize that the axis of the phylogenetic rotation of the complex seems to coincide with the physiologic rotational axis. That would certainly have been an advantage, since it permitted the complex to slowly rotate during the evolution, without impairing its hearing function. The articulation between malleus and incus is well developed in all cetaceans and the malleus is strongly fused with the tympanic bone.

In one group of cetaceans the tympanic membrane has been replaced by the bony tympanic plate. *Kogia,* as an example, has a very specialized malleus-incus complex. The transversal part is missing along with the tympanic ligament, but the fusion between the gonial and the tympanic bone is still strong. An analysis reveals, however, the apparent absence of a rotational axis of the malleus-incus complex, thus making this group and exception among mammals. The short arm of the incus is strong and has a flat contact with the periotic (Fig. 15). Mainly because the transversal part of the malleus is not developed. the center of mass of the complex is in the region of the articulation and thus rather central (Fig. 12, F).

The malleus-incus complex in bats has two rotational axes, and two modes of vibration (Figs. 13 and 14). Although the situation is not too clear, the cetaceans

non-rotational mode in Cetacea

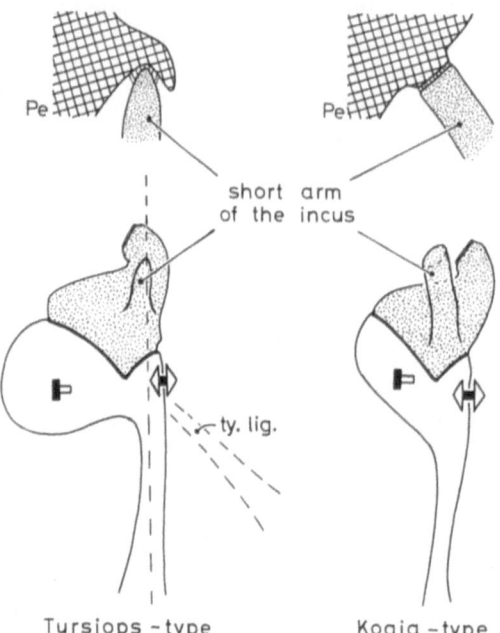

Pe

Pe

short arm
of the incus

ty. lig.

Tursiops – type          Kogia – type

Fig. 15. Semi-schematic section through the malleus-incus complex in cetaceans, along with details of the anchoring of the short arm of the incus. Especially in the *Kogia*-type the vibratory mode indicated by the *double arrow* seems to be important (no rotational axis!)

possibly also have two different modes of vibration, as far as the complex is concerned. The basic one for the *Tursiops*-type is the rotation around the axis shown in Fig. 12. A semi-schematic section through such a malleus-incus unit, parallel to the rotational axis and thus perpendicular to the transversal part, reveals the cylindrical transversal part to be supported on one side only by the gonial (*left side* of Fig. 15). During hearing the gonial may bend, as indicated by the *double arrow*. Such a motion would push the stapes in and out of the oval window. In the *Tursiops*-type this sort of motion seems to be suppressed by the anchoring of the short arm of the incus in the pit of the periotic, as indicated in the section at the top.

No morphologic axis of rotation is developed in the *Kogia*-type and probably because of this the short arm of the incus has a broad contact with the periotic, somewhat aside from the direction of the gonial. The gonial appears to be reasonably free to bend, causing motions indicated by the *double arrow*. To be sure, this has not been demonstrated, but it seems a likely mechanism. If so, the *Kogia*-type would primarily vibrate in a way which is, to a lesser degree, also present in the *Tursiops*-type. Therefore, a gradual change from the *Tursiops*-type to the *Kogia*-type during the evolution would cause no major troubles for the mechanism of the malleus-incus complex. Whatever the details, the extremely specialized ear in *Kogia* and similar forms needs special attention. As far as malleus and incus are concerned, this is undoubtedly the most highly specialized ear among mammals.

So far the three main lines of evolutionary radiation have been described, with emphasis on the various details. To demonstrate how great the differences can be, two ossicular chains of comparable size will be contrasted. One is of the freely mobile type,

two specialized forms of the ossicular chain

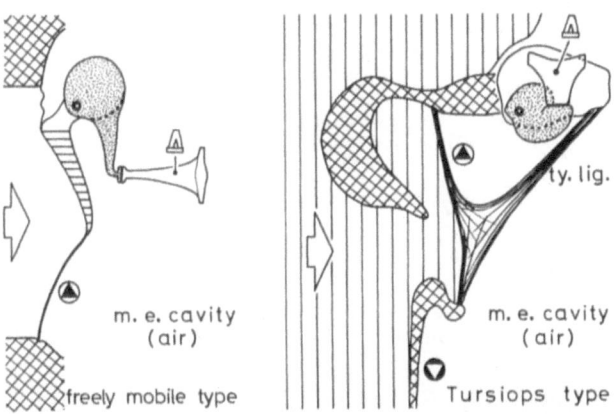

Fig. 16. Two of the larger ossicular chains seen directly along the axis of rotation (*hollow circle*). The manubrium is *hatched* and the incus *stippled*. In the low-frequency form (*left*) the ossicles are rodlike, but in the high-frequency form (*right*) they are extremely compact and thus insensitive to mechanical resonances of their components. ty. lig.: tympanic ligament

similar to the human ear, and as such a low-frequency form. The other is the ossicular chain of a dolphin, specialized for high ultrasonic sound (Fig. 16). In both cases we look directly along the rotational axis and from the side of the incus. Thus, we see the projection of the ossicular chain onto a plane perpendicular to the rotational axis. The latter is marked by a *hollow dot*. The manubrium of the malleus is *hatched* in Fig. 16 and Fig. 17 to facilitate comparison. The two forms in Fig. 16 show several conspicuous differences. The ossicular chain in the freely mobile type contains many rodlike components: the manubrium of the malleus, the long arm of the incus, and the crura of the stapes. Such a construction is adequate for lower frequencies. At high frequencies all these long and slender structures will vibrate, relative to each other, in the fundamental frequency, as well as in higher modes. In other words, the ossicular chain does not then act as a rigid system any more, instead these intra-ossicular vibrations will greatly increase the nonlinearity of the ear. Furthermore, if the parts of the ossicles vibrate relative to each other, the entire chain becomes increasingly ineffective as an apparatus for conducting sound.

If the components are small, as they are in bats, they are still stable at high frequencies. Troublesome are only the large ears, which have to be able to transmit mechanically the high-frequency vibrations to the inner ear. Dolphins are thus a perfect example, since they are the only mammals with large middle ears that are sensitive to high ultrasonic sound. In *Tursiops* the greatest sensitivity of the ear is at ~50 kHz - 70 kHz, according to Johnson (1966). Extraordinary measures have been taken to suppress the vibration of parts of ossicles, relative to each other, and that is why the ossicular chain deviates so much from that in other mammals (Fig. 16). At first, glance we see that no rodlike components are present. The manubrium has been lost, so that this source of mechanical noise is removed. The transversal part has almost the shape of a bean, and it is therefore extremely rigid and not prone to vibrate. A comparinson of the incus in both forms (see also Fig. 15) shows that the long arm in dolphins is tremendously stout and compact, so that vibrations of its parts become very unlikely. The stapes, last but not least, is quite conical, with both crura normally entirely fused together

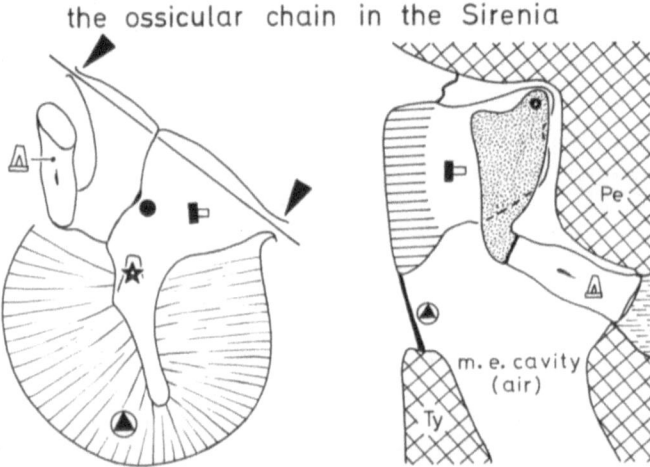

Fig. 17. The malleus-incus complex in the sirenian ear is an extraordinarily clear arrangement, because the rotational axis is solidly fused at both ends (*left*). A view directly along the rotational axis (*right*) shows the mechanics to be similar to the ones shown in Fig. 16. Sirenians have a modified transitional type of the malleus-incus complex; see also Fig. 8, *B*. The manubrium is hatched and the incus is stippled

and therefore truly stable. Mechanical stability of the ossicles is still increased by the fact that they are composed of very dense, ceramiclike bone. Despite the mechanical stability of the ossicles, they are nevertheless separated by well-developed articulations, indicating that some motions occur between the ossicles. Reasons for the development of the tympanic ligament have already been discussed earlier.

Manatees have a special modification of the transitional type (Fig. 17). They are of special interest because their ear is built in a clear and straightforward manner without all the peculiarities that make the cetacean ear so complicated. The malleus-incus complex is fused with the periotic at the side of the incus and with the tympanic at the side of the gonial (see also Fig. 5). On the *right side* of Fig. 17 the complex is presented as seen along the rotational axis, so that it is directly comparable to Fig. 16. Obviously the center of mass is outside the axis; in basic mechanics it is remarkably similar to the freely mobile type. Despite the firm anchoring of the complex, well-developed articulations are seen between the ossicles. Such a fusion of the complex cannot be interpreted as an impairment of hearing. These animals emit their well-known songs probably as a means of acoustic communication or acoustic contact. They are within the audible range of man, according to the measurements of Schevill (1965).

In summary, the malleus-incus complex has three basic lines of evolutionary adaptation. They differ primarily in the rigidity of the anchoring of the complex, the mass, and distribution of the mass relative to the rotational axis. In the *Kogia*-type ear no rotational axis is developed. The natural frequency of the rotating system is mainly governed by the torsional stiffness of the anchoring system and by the moment of inertia. The latter, in turn, is varied by changes in the distribution of the mass, according to Steiner's Satz (parallel-axis theorem). In nearly all species a well-developed articulation between malleus and incus occurs, the marine mammals with their heavy, fused malleus being no exception. Only in a number of forms with a freely mobile type does a fusion between malleus and incus take place.

# 7. Stapes Complex

At the inner end of the mammalian middle ear resides the stapes, the footplate of which drives the liquid of the inner ear. The motions of this footplate are, therefore, of critical importance for hearing. All mammals have a stapes that is separated from the malleus-incus complex by a thin layer of cartilage or other soft tissues. Therefore the stapes complex is a semi-independent part of the ossicular chain. It consists of the stapes, the annular ligament, and the stapedial muscle; the latter will be discussed in connection with the tensor tympanic muscle later.

The stapes complex is essentially a simple mass-spring system (Fig. 18). Mass is represented by the bony stapes, while the spring is localized in the anchoring of the stapes, i. e., in the annular ligament. Such an arrangement will vibrate in a pistonlike manner. However, its amplitudes at physiologic sound pressures are submicroscopically small and thus hard to determine. Békésy (1936) described a variety of stapedial motions in human cadavers, but improved technology revealed that the motion of the footplate is basically pistonlike, even at high sound pressures (Hogmoen and Gundersen, 1977).

Contrary to the statements in some books and textbooks, the stapes is not fused with the periotic in any of the mammalian species, cetaceans included. Instead, the stapes is held in place in the oval window (Fenestra vestibuli) by the annular ligament. This ligament has the form of a belt and is predominantly composed of fibres running in radial direction, thus bridging the circular gap between the footplate of the stapes and the circumference of the oval window. Great differences in thickness and width exist between the various species. Thickness is the distance from the inner ear margin to the middle ear margin, while width is the extension in axial-radial direction (*lower right*). Because of the orientation of the fibers, the stiffness of the anchoring of the stapes increases with increasing thickness of the annular ligament but decreases with increasing width. Hence, in ears where the stapes is firmly held the annular ligament has a small width but a great thickness. This is the case in many marine mammals, especially dolphins. Where the stapes is not anchored firmly, for example in the moles (*Talpa*), the mole rats (*Spalax*), the sloths (*Bradypus*), the elephants, and many others, the annular ligament usually is not thick but wide.

A simple mass-spring system has a natural frequency that depends on the spring constant (the stiffness) and the mass of the vibrating body. The mass of the spring will be ignored and it is assumed that the reference mass is large enough to be considered immobile for all practical purposes. Besides the elasticity, the annular ligament will certainly have internal friction so that the stapes complex is a highly dampened arrangement. For purposes of simplification, the dampening has been omitted in Fig. 18, but is included in Fig. 24, which shows the mechanical analogs. Since the stapes complex is a vibrating system with its own frequency characteristic, even in the absence of the malleus-incus complex, it can truly be considered a semi-independent subsystem of the mammalian middle ear.

The stapedial artery in ancestral mammals ran through the stapes, certainly one of the reasons for mammals developing a stapes in the form of a stirrup. Phylogenetically the stapedial artery is a very old structure (Goodrich, 1930). But as the animals phylogenetically increased in size this artery was gradually replaced by other vessels (Tandler 1902), because the opening between the two crura became too narrow for an enlarged vessel, as mentioned previously. The majority of modern mammals lacks the stapedial

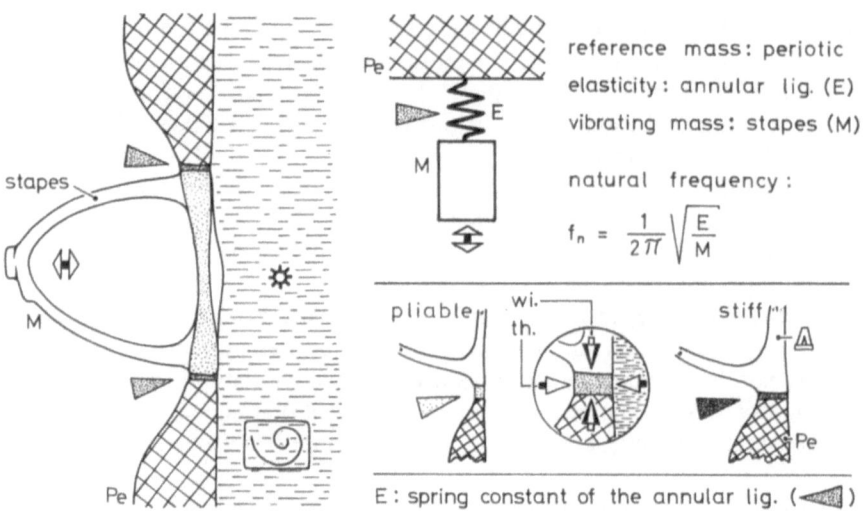

Fig. 18. Basic construction of the stapes complex. The *arrows* indicating the elastic element point towards the annular ligament. *th.:* thickness; *wi.:* width of the annular ligament, as shown in the enlargement. Basically, the stapes complex is a simple mass-spring system. See also Fig. 19

artery, but they nevertheless retain the form of a stirrup for their stapes. This might be for purely historical reasons, but more seems involved. In Fig. 19 the columella in birds is contrasted with the stapes in mammals. In both cases the footplate (the clipeolus in birds) is held at its circumference by the annular ligament, which represents an elastic element. It is drawn as a spring in the schematic illustration on top. The driving force ($F$) acts on on one side this element, arising from the long arm of the incus in mammals. This force in birds acts more or less on the center of the clipeolus. The possibility of the clipeolus bending arises because the counteracting force is supplied by the annular ligament and thus acts upon the perimeter of the clipeolus and not upon its center. The situation in mammals is different. The force ($F$) is applied to the head of the stapes, but then it is directly applied to the circumference by the two crura. Thus, the force is directed immediately to the annular ligament, which increases the stability of the stapes. Furthermore, at the two sides of the footplate where the crura are attached, the annular ligament is often much thicker than in between (Fig. 19). In other words, the spring is strengthened where the force is applied. While this makes sense from the aspect of engineering, it creates difficulties determining both width and thickness of the ligament, because both may vary along the perimeter of the footplate. In any case, the stirrup form of the mammalian stapes represents an advantage, because the force applied by the incus is directed at the circumference and thus to the elastic element, the annular ligament.

As usual there are some exceptions. The monotremes *Ornithorhynchus* (platypus) as well as *Tachyglossus* (spiny anteater) have a columellalike stapes, but they may not be true mammals. However some mammals returned secondarily to a columellalike stapes. This happened in the marsupial mole (*Notoryctes*), in the pangolin (*Manis*), and at least two other genera seem to be well on their way in doing so, one being the tree sloth (*Bradypus*) and the other, one of the African mole rats (*Heliophobius*). All these

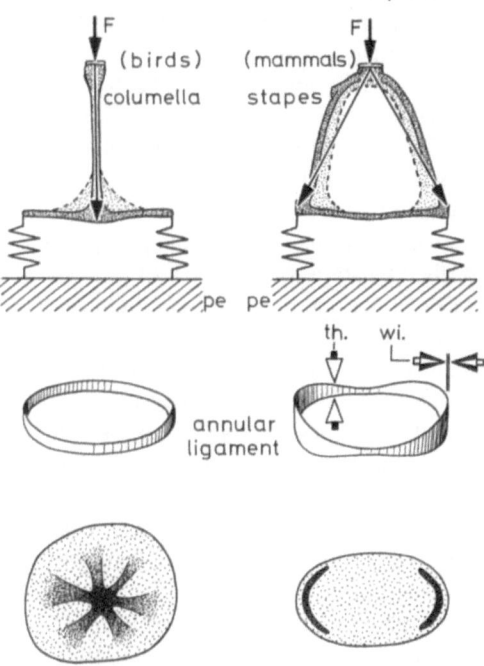

## columella versus stapes

Fig. 19. Comparison between columella and stapes. The footplate and the attachment of the stem or the crura are shown *below*. The form of the stapes is mechanically superior, because a force applied to its head is directed to the elastic element by the two crura. Thus, in most mammalian species the annular ligament is strengthened where the crura of the stapes are attached to the footplate. *th.*: thickness; *wi.*: width of the annular ligament; see also Fig. 18

forms are slow and/or subterraneous and thus do not need highly developed sensory organs. Apart from the monotremes, *Manis* and *Bradypus* may even be called living fossils. All this shows that advanced and successful mammals have a stirruplike stapes and that only some forms in small ecologic niches may secondarily return to a columellalike stapes.

Another effect should not be confused with the return to a columella. In many marine mammals the stapes as a whole is compact and massive and in many of them the crura are so much enlarged that the intercrural foramen is nearly or entirely closed. These stapes may appear to be a columella, but contrary to the real columella shown in Fig. 19, the force applied to the head of the stapes is directed to the perimeter of the footplate and not to its center. In addition to being present in some seals, this condition is found in sirenians (Fig. 17) and cetaceans (Figs. 16 and 20).

Contrary to the enormous diversity of the malleus-incus complex, the stapes is a very conservative element; it does not show a real radiation, aside from some minor changes that have been mentioned. If the malleus-incus unit is lightly built in an animal, so is the stapes. In species with a rather massive ossicular chain, the stapes shows the same bulkiness as malleus and incus. Because the stapes complex is a simple mass-spring system, the distribution of the mass is not that important for the stapes. That is why localized balancing masses, such as the head of the malleus or the orbicular apophysis, are not developed by the mammalian stapes.

As is usually the case in mammalogy the situation in man is known best. Eysell (1970), Brunner (1954), Wolff et al. (1971), and Anson and Donaldson (1973) have thoroughly described the anchoring of the stapes in man and these are only a few of the authors who have examined this aspect. Békésy (1942) and Glaninger (1961) have measured the force necessary to extract the stapes from the human cadaver. Some of the small mammals have been examined from this aspect by Wassif (1946), Kobayashi (1955), Henson (1961), Pye and Hinchcliffe (1968), Hinchcliffe and Pye (1969), and others. Henson (1961) found that in high-frequency forms of the bats, the fibers of the annular ligament tend to be short, thus resulting in a small width. Anchoring of the stapes in some marine mammals has been described by Reysenbach de Haan (1957), McCormick et al. (1970), Ramprashad et al. (1972), Solntseva (1975), and others.

Cetaceans, especially the dolphins, pose a peculiar problem because the stapes appears immobile for all practical purposes indeed so much so that it was repeatedly described as fused with the periotic, which is by no means the case. To clarify this point Fleischer (1976c) studied the anchoring system of the stapes in cetaceans and sirenians. All were found to have annular ligaments and the area of the attachment of this ligament to both stapes and periotic to have a highly specialized microstructure.

Given that the area of the attachment of the annular ligament to the stapes is an auxiliary measure for the stiffness of the connection, several relations were determined. The area of the footplate in cetaceans is roughly equal to the area of the attachment of the annular ligament to the stapes. More importantly as the ear phylogenetically increases, the mass of the stapes increases about 12 - 16 times faster than the area of attachment of the annular ligament. Hence, it was concluded that the stapes complex is a mass-spring system, which is tuned to certain frequencies mainly by increasing or decreasing the mass of the stapes. Those species (dolphins), which are known to use a sonar system based on high ultrasonic sound, where shown to have very light stapes but a very large area of attachment. Low-frequency forms, on the other hand, have massive stapes and only a small area where the ligament is attached to it.

These relations are visualized in Fig. 20. The stapes of a high-frequency form (*upper left*) is drawn in such a way that the area of its footplate is equal to that in a low-frequency form (*upper right*). Because the attachment area and the area of the footplate are about equal, both should have the same form of the stapes, if the mass grows with the area of the attachment. This, however, is not the case the difference in shape being due to the mass increasing much faster (about 12 - 16 times) than the area of the attachment. In other words, the spring may be equal in these two cases, but the mass load is drastically increased in the low-frequency form, which, however, will result in a low natural frequency.

Despite its great importance, the anchoring of the stapes has not received much attention, so that its exact physical values are unknown. However, a variety of measurements of the middle ear apparatus have been made and usually the displacement of the stapes was measured as the output of the middle ear. Using his capacitive probe, Békésy (1941) found that the amplitude of the stapes decreases more or less steadily from ~100 Hz to 2500 Hz, the upper limit of his experimental frequency range. He also described a variety of rotations of the stapes. Other authors later arrived at different results. Guinan and Peake (1967) found that the stapes in the cat predominantly vibrates in a pistonlike mode and the same was found in human cadavers by Høgmoen and Gundersen (1977). Since no fundamental difference in the anchoring of the stapes was determined, it is assumed that this holds true for mammals in general.

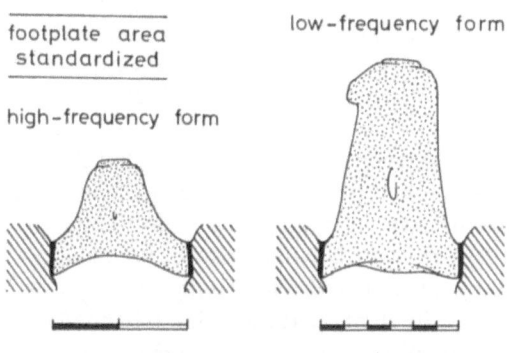

annular ligament
and mass of stapes in cetaceans

footplate area
standardized

low-frequency form

high-frequency form

allometric relations in the Cetacea:

$$\frac{\text{area (fen. vest.)}}{\text{area (ann. lig.)}} \approx 1 \qquad \frac{\Delta \text{mass (stapes)}}{\Delta \text{area (ann. lig.)}} \approx 12 \text{ to } 16$$

Fig. 20. In cetaceans the mass-spring system of the stapes complex is predominantly governed by variations of the mass. At the same size of the annular ligament the low-frequency form has a much more massive stapes than the high-frequency form. The mass of the stapes increases about 12 - 16 times faster than the area of the attachment of the annular ligament at the stapes

Physical measurements of the spring constant of the annular ligament are not available. Whereas Bekesy (1942) needed a weight of 320 g to extract the stapes from the oval window in the human cadaver, Glaninger (1961) needed only 162 - 177 g. Although this is a rather unphysiologic treatment, it nevertheless shows that the stapes can be extracted. In dolphins, for example, extraction is not possible, because the stapes is held so incredibly fast by the annular ligament. Typical low-frequency forms, such as the various types of moles, generally show wide but thin annular ligaments (see Fig. 18), indicating that the stapes is not firmly held. Probing reveals great mobility of the stapes in these forms and it is possible to extract the stapes. Monotremes also have a wide and thin ligament, not unlike those found among reptiles.

The stapes is generally the lightest element in the ossicular chain. In Figs. 3, 7, and 16 (*left side*) the stapes, seen from its narrow side, appears columellalike and heavy. From this aspect these figures may be misleading, because the crura of the stapes are normally hollow, so that the stapes is very light, while malleus and incus are quite massive. As a rule of thumb, the malleus-incus complex is normally 10 - 18 times more heavy than the stapes. The weight of the stapes in dolphins can amount to less than 5% of the combined weight of malleus and incus. This relation is of importance, because it is much easier to tune a vibrational system to high frequencies if the mass involved is small. Although the vibrational mode is different, it may be assumed that the stapes complex has a natural frequency above that of the malleus-incus complex. More functional details will be discussed in connection with the middle ear morphology and the frequency response of the ear.

# 8. Middle Ear Muscles and Articulations

The two middle ear muscles are fundamental components of the mammalian hearing apparatus. One is the stapedial muscle, which is attached to the stapes near its head, and the other is the tensor tympani muscle, which is attached to the malleus at various places depending on the type of malleus-incus complex. The basic arrangement, as found in the ancestral type, is shown in Fig. 21. While nearly all mammals examined thus far have both muscles developed to a greater or lesser degree, nevertheless some exceptions were found. The stapedial muscle is missing in the monotremes, but the tensor tympani is developed. The opposite was found true of the pangolin (*Manis*); the tensor tympani muscle is missing, while the stapedial muscle is present. In this species the presence of a cavernous blood sponge at the circumference of the tympanic membrane may have somethin to do with the missing tensor tympani.

Contraction of the stapedial muscle pulls at the stapes perpendicular to its footplate-head direction. Thus, the general direction of the force applied to the stapes by this muscle is almost parallel to the plane of the footplate. (Actually it is parallel to the plane of the annular ligament, because in many species the footplate is not flat, but either bulges outward, as in the weasel (*Mustela*), or bulges inward as shown in Fig. 20 for the dolphins.) Because of this, the stapedial muscle forces one side of the footplate into the vestibulum, while the opposite side is pulled outward, toward the middle ear. In other words, the muscle acts upon the spring represented by the annular ligament.

The footplate of the mammalian stapes is oval or bean-shaped, as in man. In any case the footplate is elongated, thus having a long and a short axis. In most species the stapes muscles pulls the stapes in a direction more or less parallel to the long axis of the footplate. Because of the phylogenetic rotation of the malleus-incus complex already described in cetaceans, the stapedial muscle pulls obliquely or even perpendicularly to the long axis of the footplate in these animals.

The stapedial muscle originates in a groove of the periotic and thus has the same reference mass as the stapes itself. In most species the facial nerve runs along the bottom of the groove, so normally the stapedial muscle originates in part at the perineurium of the facial nerve. It does not matter whether the muscle is weak or strong. Only in some species, such as man, is the stapedial muscle enclosed by a bony cover. This situation seems to be characteristic for low-frequency forms. In high-frequency forms, such as bats or dolphins, the stapedial muscle is very large and often really onion-shape, indicating great strength. The muscle in these species is not covered by a bony housing.

Through action of the stapedial muscle the stapes can be tilted somewhat; for this reason the articulation between incus and stapes has to allow for some lateral give. Probing of this connection reveals that this is the case and also that the articulation is comparatively weak, thus making it possible to separate the stapes from the malleus-incus unit. The contact area between incus and stapes is a flat piece of cartilage or other soft tissue and the capsule around the articulation is not strong.

Furthermore, at the end of the long arm of the incus is the lenticular process, which in turn forms the articulation together with the head of the stapes (see Fig. 3). The lenticular process is not unlike a mushroom, the stem of which is attached to the long arm of the incus, while the cap is in contact with the stapes. This area of the lenticular process is shown at the tip of the long arm of the incus in Figs. 8 and 10, among others. Due to this lenticular process there is also some lateral give in the ossicular chain. Such

## middle ear muscles

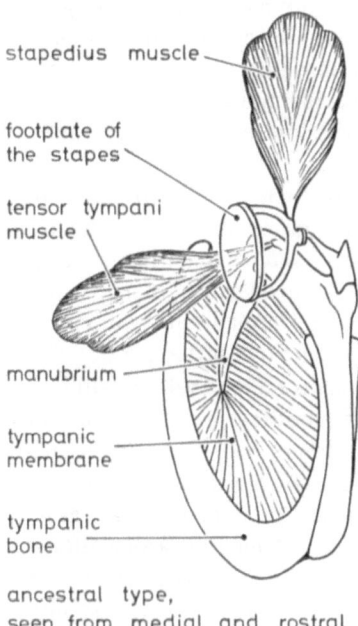

stapedius muscle

footplate of
the stapes

tensor tympani
muscle

manubrium

tympanic
membrane

tympanic
bone

ancestral type,
seen from medial and rostral

Fig. 21. Relation between the ossicular chain and the two middle ear muscles (as shown for the ancestral type). Basically the forces applied by the muscles have directions almost perpendicular to each other; see also Fig. 1, *B*

a process, however, is not indispensable, because it is not developed where the ossicles are stout and massive, as in the cetaceans and the sirenians.

All mammals have such a soft connection between stapes and incus which makes the stapes complex a semi-independent vibrating system. Of course, the connection is an elastic element, the stiffness of which influences the vibration of the ossicular chain. No physical measurements of the spring constant of these connections have been made. But it is certain that this stiffness is small, compared to that of the annular ligament, at least in those species with a stapes anchored very firmly by the annular ligament.

The second middle ear muscle, the tensor tympani muscle, pulls the malleus inside almost perpendicular to the tympanic membrane (Fig. 21). Therefore its purpose was always assumed to be the increase of tension in the tympanic membrane. Undoubtedly the contraction of this muscle increases the tension of the membrane, but this may be only one of the effects involved. This can be concluded from the fact that in the *Kogia*-type middle ear, which lacks a tympanic membrane, nevertheless a well-developed tensor tympani muscle is present. In a system so ingeniously designed, anything is omitted that is not useful, e. g., the transversal part of the malleus in the *Kogia*-type and many other examples.

Figure 21 shows that the action of the tensor tympani would push the stapes into the vestibulum, if this were not impeded by the stapedial muscle. But in any case the tensor tympani tightens both articulartions of the ossicular chain. The incus-stapes connection is compressed, while the malleus-incus articulation is wrenched. The latter effect is enhanced by the ligamentous capsule around the articulation holding both surfaces together. In a regular spring the spring constant does not change if the spring is compressed or extended within its linear range. But because the ear is such a complicated arrangement the spring constants of these articulations may well change due to the muscle's action. Experimental data are not available. Helmholtz (1868) expressed the opinion that the contractions of the middle ear muscles prevent clattering of the ossicular chain at high frequencies.

At this point some details of the connections of the ossicular chain are mentioned. The internal surface of a regular malleus-incus articulation has a shape of a V, the incus having the wedge and the malleus having the notch (Figs. 1 and 8). In the microtype the wedge forms an angle of ~ 90°, while the angle increases in many freely mobile types; the relief of the internal surface is smaller in the latter case. Normally the two surfaces are not flat, but somewhat rounded to resemble a saddle. The two surfaces inside the articulations in cetaceans are quite different (Fig. 15); one is rather small; the other, larger. The sirenian ear has a malleus-incus articulation with both surfaces rather flat and of about equal area. That these animals have such an articulation at all is amazing, given the fact that their malleus is so tightly fused with the tympanic. This has to be of functional significance, because otherwise it would have been reduced. Although cetaceans as well as sirenians lost their hind limbs entirely, they nevertheless retained the articulations of their ossicular chain. In some rodents, such as the chinchilla, malleus and incus are fused in the adult yet hearing is excellent. In the African mole rat, *Heliophobius,* not only the articulation is fused, but also most of the long arm of the incus is fused with the malleus. This may indicate that hearing in such specialized species as *Heliophobius,* which never come out of the ground throughout their life, is not of great importance. As a general rule the malleus-incus articulation is well developed in all forms with a malleus solidly fused with the tympanic bone. The normal articulation can be replaced in some species by a bony fusion, but this seems to occur only in the freely mobile type.

Another point of interest is the size of both articulations of the ossicular chain. The malleus-incus articulation is always much larger than the incus-stapes articulation. Although no detailed measurements have been made it is estimated that the area of the malleus-incus articulation ~ 15 to 50 times larger than the area of the incus-stapes articulation. This depends on, among other factors, whether or not the malleus has a "head," as in man.

The evolutionary radiation of the malleus-incus complex also effects the middle ear muscles (Fig. 22). Although with some variation, the attachments of both middle ear muscles are almost opposite to each other in the terrestrial forms (*A* through *D*). In the ancestral type and in the microtype, (*A* and *D*), the tensor tympani is attached to the malleus at the end of the transversal part. During the changes leading to the freely mobile type (*A* through *C*) the attachment of the tensor gradually shifts down onto the manubrium of the malleus. In man and some other species the tensor is attached somewhat closer to the rotational axis than is the stapedial muscle. The exact opposite is true in the *Tursiops*-type (*E*). Here the attachment of the tensor is farther from the rotational axis than that of the stapedial muscle. Only initially does the situation seem to differ from that in terrestrial forms. Things look different because of the evolutionary rotation of the malleus-incus complex. The tensor tympani muscle is attached to the malleus at the opposite side from the tympanic ligament; Fig. 16 may help to understand the arrangement. Basically both muscles act in the same way, relative to each other and to the rotational axis, as in the terrestrial forms.

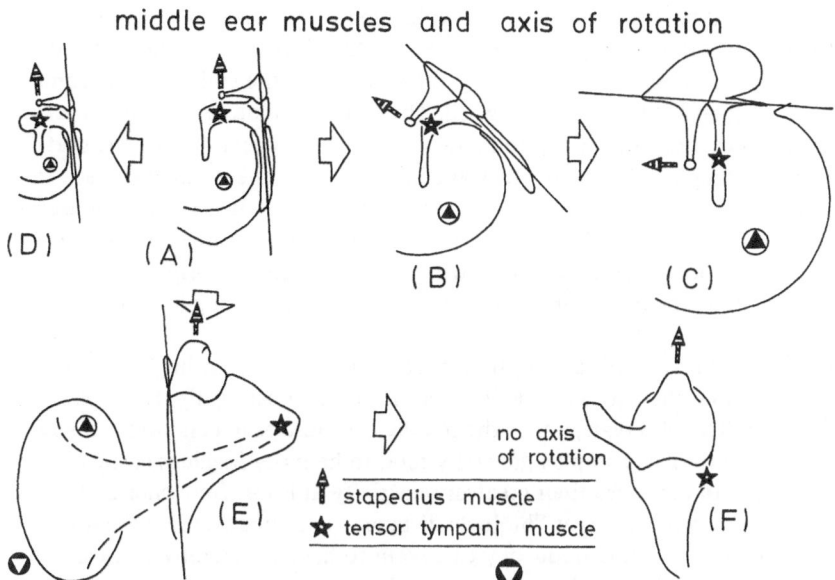

(D)    (A)    (B)    (C)

no axis
of rotation
―――――――――――――
↑ stapedius muscle
★ tensor tympani muscle

(E)    (F)

Fig. 22. Radiation of the malleus-incus complex, with special emphasis on the attachments of the middle ear muscles. The relation between the muscle attachments and the rotational axis remains remarkably constant. In the *Kogia*-type (*F*) the tensor tympani muscle is well developed although no tympanic membrane is present. The capital letters refer to the types defined in Fig. 8 and referred to in Figs. 10 and 12

A peculiar situation is found in the *Kogia*-type ear (Fig. 22, *F*). No tympanic membrane is developed, but nevertheless a tensor tympani muscle is present. Since the transversal part is also gone, the muscle is attached to the malleus just beside the articulation. Since a rotational axis of the malleus-incus complex cannot be found, the distance from the axis of both muscles cannot be determined. But both middle ear muscles apply their force in directions almost perpendicular to each other as usual.

A comparison of the various types of ears shows the tensor tympani to act in such a way as to impede rotational vibrations around the standard axis shown in Fig. 22, with the exception of the *Kogia*-type. Hence the suppression of this rotational mode can be assumed to be its main function.

Here the situation found in the microtype must be recalled. Because of the development of the orbicular apophysis this type ear has two clearly defined modes of vibration of the malleus (Figs. 13 and 14) and a second rotational axis. Of great interest is the application of the force of the tensor tympani to the malleus at, or very near, this second rotational axis. This axis is associated with the high-frequency mode of vibration and, therefore, contractions of the tensor tympani will obviously suppress the low-frequency mode but not, or only barely, the high-frequency mode. This clearly points to a selective filtering with the tensor acting as a high-pass filter. Although not clearly established, a similar vibrational mode seems to act in part in the *Tursiops*-type and predominantly in the *Kogia*-type ear.

In those ear types where the malleus is solidly fused with the tympanic, the tensor tympani muscle is usually very well developed, indicating that it is quite strong. Although no detailed measurements have been taken the tensor seems much smaller in the freely mobile type.

47

From the structural analysis as well as the evolutionary changes described, the following function of the tensor tympani muscle is deduced: it tightens the two articulations of the ossicular chain and suppresses the rotation of the malleus-incus complex around the standard axis shown in Fig. 22. The stapedial muscle acts upon the annular ligament; its action is assumed to increase the spring constant (i. e., the stiffness) of the stapes complex. Action of the stapedial muscle on the isolated stapes would thus lead to an increase of the natural frequency. If the tensor tympani muscle has the influence of a high-pass filter and the stapedial muscle increases the natural frequency of the stapes, both muscles together will alter the frequency response in such a way as to decrease the sensitivity for low frequencies, while increasing it for high frequencies.

Anatomic evidence favors this assumption, because those groups using high ultrasound for echolocation, the bats and the dolphins, have the most highly developed middle ear muscles. The observation that the middle ear muscles in ears with a freely mobile type of malleus-incus complex generally tend to be more fragile is easily explained. These types of ears have their greatest sensitivity at lower frequencies, the animals usually having a much larger "biologic distance" and thus favoring the lower frequencies. In other words, low-frequency ears seem to have comparatively weak middle ear muscles. Of course, it could also be argued that the muscles are strong where the anchoring of the ossicular chain is rigid, but this is only another view of the same phenomenon: the anchoring of the ossicular chain (especially via the gonial and the annular ligament) is rigid in high-frequency forms and pliable in low-frequency forms.

Because the middle ear muscles contract at higher sound pressure levels they are usually considered a protective mechanism for the ear for avoiding overstimulation of the cochlea. A number of biologic arguments can be made that more is involved in the middle ear muscles than just the protective function. Birds can be very noisy, especially in large numbers; nevertheless they have only one muscle in their ear, the equivalent of the stapedial muscle, without suffering any apparent damage. Mammals in general are rather quiet animals, with exceptions of course. A typical situation may be a mouse on a meadow or a fox in the forest; it is hard to imagine their having the need to protect their ears against excessive noise. Nature did not make great evolutionary efforts to adapt the ears of mammals in general to jackhammers, sirens, or jet engines. There is no protection from unexpected sound impulses, because of the latency of the aural reflexes and also no protection from prolonged noise because of the fatigue of the muscle action. Therefore it is no surprise that noise-induced hearing damage is the number-one occupational disease in practically all the industrialized countries. The suppression of the lower frequencies provides of course some sort of protection, but noise damages the human ear predominantly at $\sim 4$ kHz, i. e., at frequencies quite high for human standards (for reasons explained on p. 56).

A great number of experimental studies have been performed to determine the function of the middle ear muscles, but only a few of them will be mentioned. Basically there are two prevailing theories explaining the function of these muscles. According to the protection theory, the muscles protect the inner ear from overstimulation by excessively loud sound; the accomodation theory, on the other hand, assumes that the frequency response of the ear is changed by these muscles, in the sense of tuning. Although both sides have accumulated considerable experimental evidence, the controversy has not yet been resolved.

Helmholtz (1868) recognized that the tensor tympani in man influences the suspension of the ossicular chain, but he emphasized that the muscle action tightens the tympanic membrane. Kato (1913) studied cats and rabbits and found that higher frequencies more effectively elicite the aural reflexes than lower frequencies. He also found that the stapedial muscle tends to respond more quickly to a sound. Crowe et al. (1931), using the newly discovered cochlear microphonics, found that low frequencies in cats are attenuated by the muscles, while the transmission of high frequencies can be improved. The reflex is most easily elicited in rabbits between 2 kHz and 4 kHz, according to Lorente de No and Harris (1933). Kobrak et al. (1935) found that the muscle contraction increases with rising stimulation level. Lindsay et al. (1936) describe the stapedial muscle in man as a protective device. Wever and Bray (1937, 1942), experimenting extensively with cats, found that lower frequencies are attenuated more than higher ones, but they concluded a protective function. Bekesy (1949) also believed in the protection theory, but he assumed the muscles to have other functions as well.

Comparing the sonar system in bats to man-made radar, Hartridge (1945) argued that the muscles protect the ear against the outgoing pulses and Henson (1965) confirmed experimentally that the muscles indeed contract with every outgoing signal. At high pulse rates, however, the muscles remain contracted. But while it is hard to believe that the ear is rendered insensitive in the latter case, it is conceivable that only the low frequencies are suppressed, thus favoring the important high frequencies.

Wersäll (1958), studying the muscles in the rabbit to a great extent, collected a vast amount of information, yet did not arrive at a final conclusion as to the biologic importance of the aural reflexes. Galambos and Rupert (1959), using chronically implanted electrodes in cats, concluded that the muscles provide remarkable protection. After thorough discussion, Simmons (1964) rejected the notion of the protective function, assuming among other things that the muscles help discriminate between internal and external sources of sounds. Møller conducted several experimental studies and summarized his own research as well as the literature on the reflex (1974b). He arrived at the conclusion that among other things the muscle action reduces the transmission at frequencies below the "principal resonance frequency" of the middle ear and extends the dynamic range; also the stapedial muscle was shown to be capable of shifting the natural frequency of the stapes towards higher frequencies.

All the evidence available combined, the lower frequencies are generally recognized to be most attenuated by the middle ear muscles. Available information indicates that some gain is to be had at higher frequencies, although this is not universally accepted. These findings confirm the functional conclusions derived from the evidence shown in connection with Fig. 22.

Furthermore, the great difference between the protection theory and the accomodation theory may not exist after all. Instead, both theories seem to be simply different views of the same effect. Man, as a typical low-frequency form, (as far as mammals are concerned), tends to concentrate on the low frequencies during experimentation and reasoning. Since low frequencies are certainly suppressed by the middle ear muscles, it is easy to justify the protection theory. In nature the high frequencies are very important, especially since they carry a lot more information than the lower ones. If an animal is concentrating on some sound-emitting target, it is useful to suppress the lower frequencies and if possible increase the sensitivity to the high frequencies. Noise from a biologic environment, as well as from inside the body (circulation, motions), occurs predominantly at lower frequencies, if only because the higher ones have been lost by atmospheric or other attenuation. When the muscle action is considered from this aspect, accomodation seems to take place. Besides reducing the noise, another important effect of the suppression of low frequencies is that loud low-frequency sounds mask weaker sounds of higher frequencies, but not vice versa (Zwicker und Feldtkeller, 1967). To avoid this cochlear effect, the low frequencies have to be attenuated for the important higher frequencies to be perceived.

The need for a good reception of high frequencies is greatest in those forms with a sonar system (sound navigation and ranging) based on ultrasonic sound. Therefore it is not surprising that bats and dolphins have exceptionally well-developed middle ear muscles. In typical low-frequency forms the reception of high frequencies is not greatly needed; thus, their muscles tend to be much weaker. It is conceivable that in some of these species that never come out of the ground, the muscles may be partially or even entirely reduced. The middle ear muscles in man, a normal low-frequency species, are not really typical for mammals in general.

# 9. Audiogram and Middle Ear Construction

To repeat man is a low-frequency form among mammals. The hearing capabilities in man were thoroughly examined by Fletcher and Munson (1933), using a large number of test subjects; a number of later studies confirmed their results on the frequency response of the human ear. Sensitivity is greatest in the frequency range of 3 kHz to 4 kHz; the upper limit of hearing is at ~ 20 kHz in children, but decreases with age toward presbycusis. Thus, for adults the upper limit of hearing is at ~ 15 kHz. Although the methods employed to determine the hearing capabilities in mammalian animals are widely different and both direct and indirect, it is nevertheless clear that only a few species do not have a hearing range extending into the range of ultrasound (frequencies above 20 kHz). One such indirect method was worked out by Fleischer (1973a, 1976a, 1976b), who demonstrated that the structure of the inner ear — especially the suspension system of the basilar membrane — depends on the hearing capability. From all the results available, elephants, camels, perhaps sloths, and various forms of moles apparently have similar, low-frequency characteristics of their ears. All of these species have a freely mobile type of the malleus-incus complex and tympanic membranes larger than those of others with comparable size of the inner ear.

The primates have a freely mobile type of the malleus-incus unit or at least a transitional type. As expected, they tend to be low-frequency animals and the frequency of the greatest sensitivity decreases with increasing size of the ear. The hearing acuity in the chimpanzee (*Pan*) is quite simimar to that in man, according to Elder (1934). Wendt (1934) studied some old-world monkeys and found that their hearing range extends somewhat beyond the upper frequency limit in man. According to Stebbins (1973), the hearing range in Cercopithecinae extends up to ~ 40 kHz with the best sensitivity at 8 kHz. Vernon (1967) discussed the problems involved with hearing research in primates. Tree shrews (*Tupaia*) and bush babies (*Galago*) have been examined by Heffner et al. (1969a, b); according to these tests their range of greatest sensitivity extends up to 16 kHz.

The small desert-dwellers with the enlarged middle ear cavity and the freely mobile malleus-incus complex have remarkable sensitivity at low frequencies. Fink and So-fouglu (1966) examined the Mongolian gerbil (*Meriones*), Vernon et al. (1971) studied the kangaroo rat (*Dipodomys*), while the chinchilla (*Chinchilla*) was tested by Strother (1967) and Miller (1970).

Other small species, but with an ear in which the malleus is fused firmly with the tympanic, have a drastically different hearing capability. Crowley et al. (1965) found that the laboratory rat (*Rattus*) has the greatest sensitivity at ∼ 40 kHz and seems to hear up to 100 kHz. Zippelius und Schleidt (1956), Smith (1975), and others found that young mice communicate with their mothers by high ultrasonic sounds. Dice and Barto (1952) determined that one of these, *Peromyscus*, hears frequencies up to 100 kHz. All these rodents have at least a small orbicular apophysis thus demonstrating that this additional mass is not detrimental to hearing, at least not for high-frequency forms. Only a very few of the great number of studies on the hearing capabilities can be mentioned, particularly as far as bats (Microchiroptera) are concerned. Their echo-location system was discovered several times independently and was described by Griffin (1958), the grand master of bat research. As previously mentioned, bats have a well-developed orbicular apophysis and more or less all of them may hear up to frequencies of 100 kHz or more.

Audiograms or equivalents from bats have been reported by Dalland (1965), Vernon and Peterson (1966), Vernon et al. (1966), and Suga (1973). Because of their auditory specialization, the audiograms represent strong cochlear and neural specializations, as shown by Neuweiler (1970), Pollack et al. (1972), and others. Within the scope of this paper, it is only of interest that the bats are specialized for perception of high frequencies.

Dolphins are another group of mammals with a sonar system based on high ultrasonic sound. But contrary to the bats, their inner ears are large and they had to solve the problems involved with hearing under water. Johnson (1966) showed that the best frequency range in the bottle-nosed dolphin (*Tursiops*) is between 50 kHz and 70 kHz; Jacobs and Hall (1972) found the greatest sensitivity in the freshwater dolphin (*Inia*) at 75 - 90 kHz. The killer whales (*Orcinus*) seem to be less sensitive to high frequencies, their greatestrange of sensitivity determined by Hall and Johnson (1972) to be at ∼ 15 kHz. More details on problems related to hearing in dolphins can be found in Kellogg (1965), Norris (1966), Diercks (1972), Evans (1973), Fleischer (1976c), among others.

The huge mysticetes are a special case because of tremendous experimental problems. Although audiograms are not available, a number of recordings of their sound emission clearly indicate that they are specialized for low and extremely low frequencies. Such recordings have been made by Schevill et al. (1964), Perkins (1966), Cummings et al. (1968, 1972), Cummings and Thompson (1971), Payne and McVay (1971), Winn et al. (1971), and others. Analysis of the structure of their inner ear confirmed their specialization for perception of very low frequencies (Fleischer, 1976a). Sirenian calls, studied by Schevill (1965), are known to be within the frequency range of the human ear.

Another aspect to be mentioned is domestication. Like all the other animals domesticated forms have the need to adapt to their environment. Sensory requirements of a poodle living in a small apartment or a rabbit living in a cage are certainly drastically different from those of their wild ancestral forms. Hence it is not surprising that domesticated animals can have rather different hearing acuities than wild specimens of the same species. Of course, this makes it troublesome to compare experimental results derived from domesticated forms. Problems of this nature have been discussed by Herre (1953), Herre und Röhrs (1971), Fleischer (1973a), among many others, and was also mentioned by Smith (1975).

The methods to determine mammalian audiograms have been reviewed by Francis (1975), and though monotremes have been neglected to a certain extent in this paper, it should be mentioned that a cochlear microphonic audiogram of the platypus (*Ornithorhynchus*) was determined by Gates et al. (1974). They found that the maximal sensitivity was at 5 kHz and concluded that the auditory system in the platypus is intermediary between that of reptiles and mammals.

This paper emphasizes that the malleus-incus complex is a rotational system. This opinion is not new, of course, as regards mammals with a configuration of the ossicular chain similar to that in man. Typical examples are guinea pigs, chinchillas, rabbits, and to some extent cats. Needless to say they are characterized by the freely mobile type or at least something very similar. Helmholtz (1868) discussed the rotational motion in man to a great extent, but in the end he settled for a one-arm lever system with the hinge at the end of the short arm of the incus. In his extensive mathematical modeling, Frank (1923) assumed the same rotational axis as was shown in this paper. This opinion was also expressed by Dahmann (1929, 1930). Bárány (1938) pointed out that in man both ossicles together are nearly balanced, relative to the rotational axis, because of the development of the head of the malleus. Some years later Békésy (1941) also adopted this opinion, as did Wever and Lawrence (1954), and a great many others. This finding appears to be generally accepted today.

Mammals with an ossicular chain very much different from that in man received only limited attention. Reysenbach de Haan (1957) and Purves (1966) assumed a rotational axis in cetaceans. Purves described a mechanism for amplifying displacement by the rotational system, something which appears to be a minor by-product of the evolutionary rotation discussed.

One purpose of this paper is to show that the malleus-incus complex is a rotating system in all therian mammals, except for the *Kogia*-type in dolphins. Furthermore, it will be demonstrated that the evolutionary radiation of the complex, as worked out by Fleischer (1973a), is caused mainly by shifting the center of mass by means of additional bony masses. The head of the human malleus is accordingly only one example of these balancing (or imbalancing) masses and thus is theoretically equivalent to the orbicular apophysis in the microtype. Connected with alterations of the torsional stiffness of the anchoring system, the shifting of the center of mass governs the natural frequency of this subsystem. The underlying physical principle is stated by the Steiner'-scher Satz, i. e., by the parallel-axis theorem. The stapes complex is another subsystem, semi-independent of the malleus-incus complex.

Although extremely specialized, the ears of cetaceans will be used to summarize the various subsystems as well as their relation to each other. This is justified because these ears also include the components and subsystems of ordinary terrestrial species. A schematic overview is presented in Fig. 23, using somewhat idealized components to illustrate the vibrational modes. In the sirenians the parts are different in appearance, yet the basic principles are the same as in the whales and dolphins.

The entire hearing organ is decoupled from the skull, i. e., it is connected to the latter by means of elastic soft tissues. Hence, it is basically a mass-spring system with a natural frequency certainly below the lower limit of hearing. It is not used to perceive

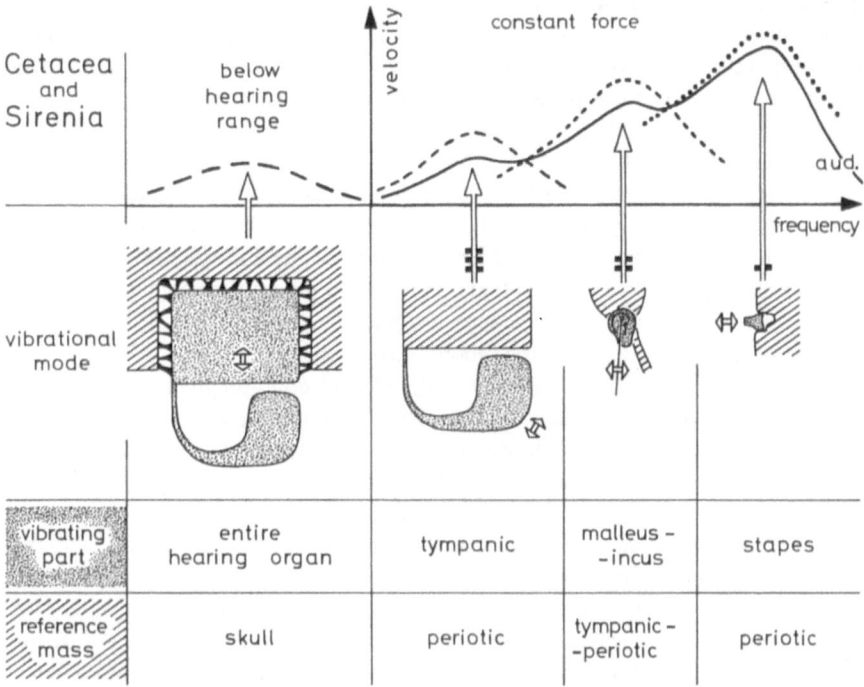

| Cetacea and Sirenia | | | | |
|---|---|---|---|---|
| **vibrating part** | entire hearing organ | tympanic | malleus – –incus | stapes |
| **reference mass** | skull | periotic | tympanic – –periotic | periotic |

Fig. 23. Semi-schematic illustration of the three subsystems of the ear in cetaceans and sirenians, as well as their influence on the audiogram (*aud.*). In terrestrial mammals only the two subsystems on the *right* are in operation. The labeling of the *arrows* referring to the subsystems is the same as in Figs. 24 and 25

sound, but on the contrary, is a mechanism to isolate both ears from each other and from the vibrations of the skull. A partial or imperfect decoupling is present in many bats, some rodents, and in seals. Nothing of this mechanism is present in man.

At somewhat higher frequencies the tympanic bone will vibrate relative to the periotic (see Fig. 5). It is, of course, a flexional mode and the "hinge" is only an aid to visualize the motion. The periotic bone has to be very massive to form a relatively stable reference mass for the tympanic. Flexional stiffness, mass, and distribution of mass govern the natural frequency of this mode. These vibrations are forced on the ossicular chain and thus stimulate the inner ear. Theoretically the mechanism can also operate in terrestrial forms with a U-shaped tympanic, but it is only effective under water, because of the matched impedances of water and soft tissues. Therefore it is assumed to be negligible in terrestrial mammals.

Next in line is the malleus-incus complex, which is a torsional system in terrestrial species and in the *Tursiops*-type among the cetaceans. As pointed out earlier there is no morphologic axis of rotation in the *Kogia*-type, rather a flexional mode of vibration is likely in these forms. In both cases the malleus-incus complex vibrates relative to both the periotic and the bulk of the tympanic bone. This complex is certainly extremely modified in cetaceans, but the functional principle is essentially the same as in man and other terrestrial mammals (see Fig. 16). It is a torsional system coupled on one side to a membrane or a membranelike receiving area for sound and on the other to the stapes. The natural frequency of the system depends on the torsional stiffness of the anchoring, as well as on mass and, most importantly, on the distribution of the mass. During the evolutionary radiation the center of mass is extensively shifted relative to the rotational axis. In this way the natural frequency can be governed effectively by varying the moment of inertia according to the Steiner'scher Satz (parallel-axis theorem).

Innermost is the stapes, which is part of a simple mass-spring system. At least in cetaceans the natural frequency of this stapes complex is governed predominantly by varying the mass, while slightly changing the spring, i. e., the annular ligament. However, observation indicates that the thickness and width of the annular ligament in other groups is also altered to a great extent. Contrary to the extensive adaptive radiation of the malleus-incus complex, the stapes complex is very conservative, all evidence indicating that it operates in a translatory mode throughout mammals.

At the *upper* part of Fig. 23 the velocity of the various components are drawn schematically with *broken lines*. Although not yet proven preliminary experimentation by the author indicates that the natural frequencies of the components follow in this order, as far as frequency is concerned. It is presented here as a concept, which can be put to the experimental test. As expected, the natural frequency rises with decreasing mass of the vibrating component. For various species these natural frequencies will be different, depending on the hearing capability.

Coupling these three subsystems together results in a very complex arrangement in which stiffness and dampening of the connections are of critical importance. Unfortunately not much is known about this except that anatomic preparation indicates the coupling connections to be relatively weak. Thus the exact response of such a system cannot be determined on this basis. However, measurement of the relative motions between footplate and periotic may yield a curve similar to the *continuous black* line in the diagram in Fig. 23. Arguments will be presented indicating that this continuous black line may represent the basic shape of the audiogram. Of course, the audiogram is customarily plotted inversely with the greatest sensitivity at the lowest point of the curve (see Fig. 25).

Mechanical equivalents of simplified middle ears will be discussed first, ignoring the influence of the tympanic membrane and the outer meatus (Fig. 24). The *marked arrows* indicate the natural frequency of the same subsystems in Figs. 23 - 25. Under these simplified circumstances, the columella in many birds or reptiles is a mass-spring system, just as the isolated stapes complex in mammals (bottom of figure). The malleus-incus complex, a torsional system, is added in mammals. Both subunits are connected elastically by means of the incus-stapes joint. Cetaceans and sirenians finally included another component into the sound-transmitting apparatus: the tympanic bone. Contrary to the other subunits it operates in a flexional mode and acts predominantly upon the rotational axis of the malleus-incus complex (see also Fig. 5). Tympanic membrane and tympanic plate are not considered, but the elasticity of the tympanic ligament is included (*top* of the figure).

Since the motions of the footplate of the stapes drive the liquids of the inner ear, it is necessary to judge the mechanical response of such simplified mechanical equivalents by the relative motions between the stapes and the reference mass. The estimated displacement of the stapes is sketched (right Fig. 24). The three subsystems in the *Tursiops*-type are predominantly connected in series therefore the greatest displacement of the stapes is expected to be caused at the natural frequency of the largest

## mechanical equivalents and displacement

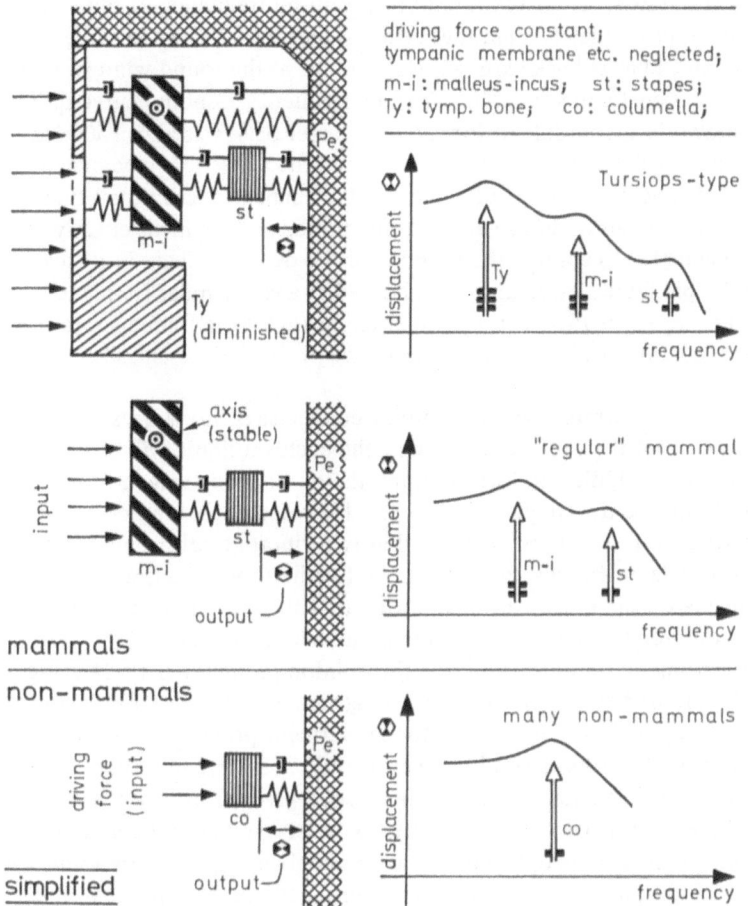

driving force constant;
tympanic membrane etc. neglected;
m-i : malleus-incus;  st : stapes;
Ty : tymp. bone;   co : columella;

Fig. 24. Simplified mechanical equivalents of three basic types of middle ears. Outer acoustic meatus, tympanic membrane, and cavity volume ignored. The frequency characteristic, especially for the *Tursiops*-type, is estimated. The more complex systems have the advantage of an enlarged bandwidth. Labeling of the arrows on the right refers to the same subsystems as in Figs. 23 and 25

component, the tympanic element. More details are not available because spring constants and the amount of dampening is unknown.

Experimentation by the author indicated that the natural frequency of the tympanic element, relative to the periotic, is at a few hundred Hz, while the greatest sensitivity of the ear is at ~70 kHz in *Tursiops,* an example of a typical dolphin. Therefore it is reasonable to assume that the displacement of the stapes is not responsible for the greatest sensitivity of the ear. Instead, the velocity of the stapes is tentatively concluded to be most relevant for the greatest sensitivity of the ear (see Fig. 23).

While the cetacean ear has three vibrating subsystem, terrestrial mammals, man included, have only two. Thus displacement curves for the stapes can be expected to be similar to the one shown in the *middle* of Fig. 24. Several measurements of this nature have been performed and although the methods varied drastically the displacement curves do show this basic shape. After experimenting with human cadavers, Onchi

(1961) concluded that there are two vibrating components in the middle ear, the malleus-incus body and the stapes. He also found that the natural frequency of the malleus-incus body is lower in frequency than that of the stapes. In 1962 Andersen et al. drove the ear of human cadavers backward, applying sound to the round window and measuring at the outer acoustic meatus. They found a frequency response curve quite similar to the one shown in the middle of Fig. 24. The larger peak was at ~ 1500 Hz and the second one at ~ 400 Hz. Møller (1963) measured the acoustic impedance in anesthetized cats and found a transfer function of similar shape. He also noted that at higher frequencies the stapes no longer follows the motions of the incus exactly. Later Guinan and Peake (1967) studied the motions of the ossicular chain in the cat by means of stroboscopic illumination and again arrived at a very similar frequency response curve of the stapes. In 1968 Rubinstein et al. measured the frequency response of the stapes in human cadavers with a capacitive probe with essentially the same results.

These experiments demonstrate that the natural frequencies of the subsystem are not altered by the liquids of the cochlea. Of course, the cochlear liquid will increase the friction of the isolated middle ear. Furthermore, the outer acoustic meatus does not seem to greatly influence the frequency response. However, these studies support the conclusion, derived from structural analysis, that two vibrating subsystems are present in the ear of terrestrial mammals, including man. Furthermore, the frequency response curves of the stapes agree with the assumption that the velocity of the stapes is most relevant for the frequency response of the entire hearing organ.

Indirect evidence from another area supports the opinion presented here. Hearing impairment caused by noise has been known for a long time to start at ~ 4 kHz; this frequency range is usually affected most when the impairment progresses. This problem and its various aspects is summarized by Dieroff (1975) and Henderson et al. (1976). Recently Bruel (1977) questioned why this is so, regardless of whether or not the persons afflicted in this way predominantly experienced high-frequency or low-frequency noise. To be sure, people working with metal and glass are predominantly exposed to high-frequency noise and they suffer much more from impairment of hearing than other occupations. But more important is the fact that the greatest sensitivity of the human ear is at ~ 4 kHz, and there is every reason to believe that the velocity of the stapes is greatest – for constant sound pressure – at that frequency. It is, of course, the natural frequency of the stapes complex in man, and therefore resonance phenomena will excessively stimulate the inner ear whenever sounds comprise strong components in the frequency range of that phenomenon. Repeated over and over again this will finally damage the inner ear irreparably. Since impairment of hearing usually develops after long periods – years or even tens of years –, exposure to many such potentially damaging events is highly likely even if the "normal" noise is not rich in such frequencies.

Displacement measurements of the stapes in cetaceans and sirenians are not available, but the audiograms are very similar to the *inverse continuous black line* in the upper part of Fig. 23. All three are highly asymmetric, the slope of the audiogram being rather gentle below the point of the maximal sensitivity and extremely steep at frequencies above that point: Johnson (1966, 1968), Jacobs and Hall (1972), and Hall and Johnson (1972). The irregularities in these audiograms at the low-frequency slope show a pattern that might be ascriped to the vibrating components, as indicated in Fig. 23. This, however, may be coincidental, and more work is necessary to clarify this relationship. Nevertheless, these audiograms support the conclusion that the cetacean middle ear consists of three subsystems in a cascading connection and also that it is the velocity of the stapes which is most relevant for the shape of the audiogram. The steep slope of the audiogram in dolphins at frequencies just above the range of greatest sensitivity results from the roll-off within all three subsystems of their middle ear.

Early in their history mammals gradually replaced the primary articulation of the lower jaw by the secondary articulation and, furthermore, they incorporated the components of the former into the sound-conducting apparatus of the middle ear. This opinion is nowadays generally accepted as the theory of Reichert and Gaupp and there is a great amount of literature dealing with this remarkable transition (Reichert, 1837; Gaupp, 1911, 1912; Crompton, 1958; Kühne, 1958; Romer, 1969; Krebs, 1975; Allin, 1975, to name only a few). Despite all these efforts the functional significance of this evolutionary transition has remained obscure, because of the fact that man's hearing capability is not that much better than that of some birds, e. g., Schwartzkopff (1968). However, man is not a typical mammal, as far as hearing is concerned, but rather a low-frequency form, compared to mammals in general. Moreover, while the great majority of mammalian species (bats and rodents combined account for roughly three-fourths of the mammalian species) is obviously very sensitive to ultrasonic sounds, no known nonmammal among vertebrates has a hearing range extending into the realm of ultrasound. This alone indicates that the mammalian hearing organ in general is superior to that of nonmammals and the incorporation of malleus and incus may have something to do with this superiority.

In connection with Figs. 23 and 24 the mammalian middle ear was previously stated to consist of semi-independent subsystems tuned to different frequencies. Since these subsystems are connected in series, the bandwidth of the entire middle ear is expanded. In other words, the additional component permits the transmission of sounds to the inner ear within a wider range of frequencies, if the system is properly engineered, and this amounts to a great biologic advantage. The principle is illustrated schematically in Fig. 25. The curved line represents the audiogram, i. e., the threshold of hearing at the various frequencies. It separates the audible range, left white, from the inaudible range.

The middle ear in "regular" terrestrial nonmammals consists of the tympanic membrane and the columella, resulting in a simple frequency-response curve. The greatest sensitivity is at the natural frequency of the columella complex. There are, of course, many deviations from such a simple system (Stellbogen, 1930; Freye-Zumpfe, 1952; Kartaschew and Iljitschow, 1964; Wever, 1968; Wever and Werner, 1970; and others). Snakes do not have a typical middle ear at all and some birds have obviously arrived at similar complex arrangements (Starck, 1960). All these special conditions will be ignored to demonstrate the basic principle.

Mammals added the malleus-incus complex, thereby expanding the bandwidth (*middle* of Fig. 25). The tone, indicated by the *square,* is shown for nonmammals in the inaudible range in the *lower part,* but as just audible in the *middle part* of Fig. 25. A corresponding gain is also present below the frequency of the maximal sensitivity due to the natural frequency of the malleus-incus complex. The audiogram represents the actual hearing capability of man or the other animals; therefore cochlear as well as neural mechanisms are also contributing elements. One factor certainly involved is the helicotrema of the inner ear which acts basically as a low-frequency shunt and will account for a great deal of the insensitivity at the very low frequencies of the

## vibrating components and audiogram

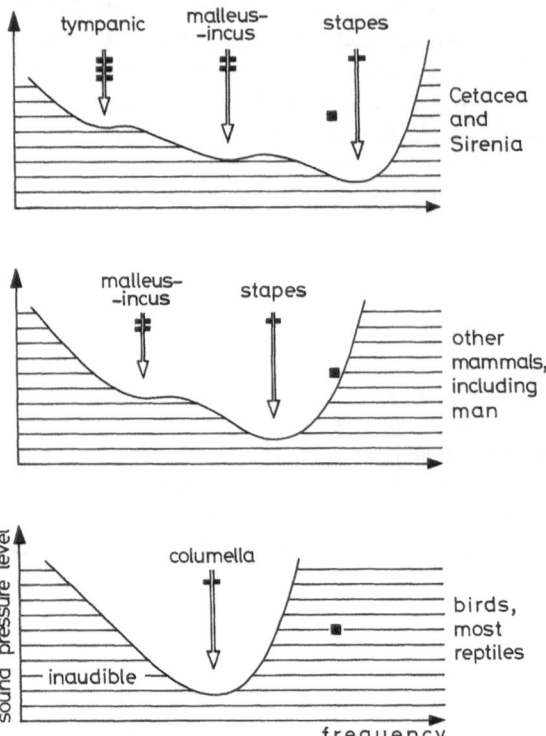

Fig. 25. Relations between the major vibrating components of the middle ear and the audiogram. Tympanic membrane and tympanic plate are omitted. The audiogram represents the threshold of hearing and it is indicated by the *curved line* which separates the inaudible area (*hatched*) from the audible field (*white*). The *dark square* represents a tone which is inaudible at the bottom, barely audible in the middle, and excellently audible at the top. The great evolutionary advantage of the more complex middle ears is an increase of the frequency range of hearing, along with the option to shape the hearing capability according to the biologic needs of the animal

hearing range. Yet the basic shape of the audiogram, including the range of the greatest sensitivity, seems to be a function of the mechanics of the middle ear.

As outlined previously, cetaceans and sirenians included another element, the tympanic bone, into the sound-transmitting system of the middle ear. Hence the bandwidth of hearing could again be expanded by adjusting the mechanics of the components. Functionally this step is equivalent to the incorporation of the malleus-incus complex in the early history of mammals. To be sure, no evidence shows that the sirenians made use of that possibility; in other words, what is known about their hearing capability and their ear does not indicate that they really extended their range of hearing.

Cetaceans, however, certainly used the theoretical chance, although the two groups did so in a different way. Odontocetes, in general, and dolphins and porpoises, in particular, are specialists for extremely high frequencies, although they can also hear very low frequencies. This group has by far the greatest frequency range of hearing in nature for which their elaborate middle ear construction is a prerequisite. The same tone, marked by a little square in Fig. 25, is therefore in the range of greatest sensitivity in the dolphin.

Mysticetes emit low and even extremely low frequencies (Schevill et al., 1964; Cummings and Thompson, 1971; and others) and the structure of their inner ear also shows that they are specialists for low frequencies (Fleischer, 1976a). Some of their calls have much of their energy concentrated at frequencies as low as 20 Hz; the question naturally arose how they manage to hear them. Barham (1973) even suggested that they use their lungs as receiver for low frequencies. Preliminary experimentation by the author showed that in the fin whale (*Balaenoptera physalus*) the natural frequency of the tympanic bone, relative to the periotic bone, is at about 30 Hz, thus making it an excellent receiver for extremely low frequencies, as indicated in Figs. 24 and 25. Since the constructional details are similar in all mysticetes, it can be concluded that all use the tympanic element as a receiver for extremely low frequencies.

So far the ear has been treated primarily as a technical measuring device and the strong influence of the physical parameters on such an extraordinarily sensitive organ is not surprising. But more is involved; although the adaptive radiation offers new advantages, it often restricts the possibilities for further specializations. Thus, there are technical, evolutionary, and environmental possibilities, as well as limitations, for specialization. All these interrelated influences and their effects on a system have been subsumed under the term *Konstruktionsmorphologie* (constructional morphology), (Weber, 1955; Seilacher, 1970). Because so many factors are involved, it is extremely difficult to use a system like the middle ear to determine phylogenetic relations between various species or groups. One thing is certain: similarity in form alone does not mean too much, because the various lines of evolutionary radiation developed independently again and again. Of course, a certain species can be excluded as ancestral to another by means of its ear structure. A freely mobile type of malleus-incus complex, for example, cannot be ancestral to a *Tursiops*-type. This can be stated with some certainty because all the evidence indicates that the evolutionary adaptation developed in the directions indicated in Fig. 8 and does not reverse itself.

This study may help to understand the underlying reasons for the evolutionary changes of the ear. But this is only one aspect and a great many more have to be considered if the evolution of mammals is to be thoroughly explained as the extensive work of Thenius (1969) showed. What is presented here is a unifying concept of structure and function of the middle ear. While some points have been more or less established, others are still awaiting the experimental test. Since the concept shows clear relations between structural details and hearing capability, its validity can be established experimentally. The relations outlined can also help gain further insight into the way of life of mammals already extinct.

## 10. Summary

As a result of structural analysis of the mammalian middle ear, the major evolutionary lines of the adaptive radiation of the ossicular chain are described. Besides this the following concept was derived.

In all species, including cetaceans, the ossicular chain is operational and the basic functional principles are the same throughout the mammals. In terrestrial forms, man included, there are two semi-independent subsystem, the stapes complex and the malleus-incus complex.

The stapes complex is a mass-spring system, with the spring represented by the annular ligament. It vibrates in a translatory mode. The malleus-incus complex is a torsional system (with the probable exception of the *Kogia*-type) and its elastic element is represented by the anchoring of the malleus and the short arm of the incus. Its natural frequency is altered by variations in the torsional stiffness and by shifting the center of mass relative to the rotational axis. The orbicular apophysis of the micro-type and the "head" of the malleus in the freely mobile type are prime examples for such imbalancing or balancing masses.

Incorporation of the malleus-incus complex into the middle ear during the early evolution of mammals resulted in an increased bandwidth of hearing and was thus a great biologic advantage. Entire groups, such as bats, dolphins, or baleen whales, might not exist the way they do, without this development.

Cetaceans and sirenians included a third vibrating element, the tympanic bone, into the sound-conducting apparatus, enabling them to further increase their frequency range of hearing.

The basic shape of the audiogram, especially the frequency range of the greatest sensitivity, is determined by the mechanics of the middle ear. Evidence shows that the velocity of the stapes is most relevant for the audiogram, and the frequency range of greatest sensitivity is defined by the natural frequency of the stapes complex.

Both middle ear muscles together are able to suppress the transmission of low frequencies, while the high frequencies are not affected or even somewhat enhanced.

*Acknowledgments.* At this point I want to express my gratitude to the great number of colleagues and friends who over the years supplied me with anatomic preparations, with equipment, space, or other help. For discussions related to the ramifications of the mechanical aspects I want to thank Dr. G. Kemper (Berlin/Bonn), and I am indebted to Prof. Dr. Dr. Duncker (Giessen) for encouragement.

# References

Airapet'yants, E., Konstantinov, A.: Echolocation in animals, 309 p. Academy of Sciences of the USSR, Leningrad (1970). Translated by: Israel Program of Scientific Translations, Jerusalem 1973

Allin, E. F.: Evolution of the mammalian middle ear. J. Morph. **147**, 403–438 (1975)

Andersen, S., Christensen, T.: Underwater sound localization in man. J. Auditory Res. **9**, 358–364 (1969)

Andersen, H., Hansen, C., Neergaard, E.: Experimental studies on sound transmission in the human ear. Acta Otolaryngol. (Stockh.) **54**, 511–520 (1962)

Anson, B., Donaldson, J.: Surgical Anatomy of the Temporal Bone and Ear. Philadelphia: Saunders p. 492

Bárány, E.: A contribution to the physiology of bone conduction. Acta Otolaryngol. (Stockh.) Suppl. **26**, 1–229, 1938

Barham, E. G.: Whales'respiratory volume as a possible resonant receiver for 20 Hz signals. Nature **245**, 220–221 (1973)

Beauregard, H.: Recherches sur l'appareil auditif chez les mammifères. J. de l'Anatomie et de la Physiologie (Paris) 366–413 (1894)

Beecher, M.: Pure-tone thresholds of the squirrel monkey (*Saimiri sciureus*). J. Acoust. Soc. Amer. **55**, 196–197 (1974)

Békésy, G. v.: Zur Physik des Mittelohres und über das Hören bei fehlerhaftem Trommelfell. Akust. Z. **1**, 13–23 (1936)

Békésy, G. v.: Über die Messung der Schwingungsamplitude der Gehörknöchelchen mittels einer kapazitiven Sonde. Akust. Z. **6**, 1–16 (1941)

Békésy, G. v.: Über die Schwingungen der Schneckentrennwand beim Präparat und Ohrenmodell. Akust. Z. **7**, 173–186 (1942)

Békésy, G. v.: The structure of the middle ear and the hearing of one's own voice by bone conduction. J. Acoust. Soc. Am. **21**, 217–232 (1949)

Békésy, G. v.: Experiments in hearing, 745 p. New York: McGraw-Hill 1960

Belkovich, M., Dubrowski, N.: Sensory fundamentals of the orientation in cetaceans. (in Russian), 204 p. Academy of Sciences of the USSR; Leningrad, 1976

Bench, R., Pye, A., Pye, J. (eds.): Sound reception in mammals, 357 p. New York: Academic Press 1975

Blauert, J.: Räumliches Hören 256 p. Stuttgart: Hirzel 1974

Boenninghaus, G.: Das Ohr des Zahnwales. Zool. Jahrbücher, Abt. Anat. **19**, 189–360 (1904)

Bruel, P.: Do we measure damaging noise correctly? Noise Control Engineering **8**, 52–60 (1977)

Brunner, H.: Attachement of the stapes to the oval window in man. Arch. Otolaryngol. **59**, 18–29 (1954)

Busnel, R.-G. (ed.): Animal Sonar Systems, Biology and Bionics. 2 Vols., p. 1233. Jouy-en-Josas, France: NATO Advanced Study Institute 1967

Cockerell, T., Miller, I., Printz, M.: The auditory ossicles of American rodents. Bull. Am. Museum, Nat. Hist., **33**, 347–380 (1914)

Crompton, A.: The cranial morphology of a new genus and species of ictidosaurian. Proc. Zool. Soc. Lond. **130**, 183–216 (1958)

Crowe, S., Hughson, W., Witting, E.: Function of the tensor tympani muscle. Arch. Otolaryngol. **14**, 575–580 (1931)

Crowley, D., Hepp-Reymond, M., Tabowitz, D., Palin, J.: Cochlear potentials in the albino rat. J. Auditory Res. **5**, 307–316 (1965)

Cummings, W., Thompson, P., Cook, R.: Underwater sounds of migrating gray whales, *Eschrichtius glaucus* (Cope). J. Acoust. Soc. Am. **44**, 1278–1281 (1968)

Cummings, W., Thompson, P.: Underwater sounds from the blue whale, *Balaenoptera musculus*. J. Acoust. Soc. Am. **50**, 1193–1198 (1971)

Cummings, W., Fish, J., Thompson, P.: Sound production and other behavior of southern right whales, *Eubalaena glacialis*. Trans. San Diego Soc. Nat. Hist. **17**, 1–14 (1972)

Dahmann, H.: Zur Physiologie des Hörens I; experimentelle Untersuchungen über die Mechanik der Gehörknöchelchenkette, sowie über deren Verhalten auf Ton und Luftdruck. Z. Hals- Nasen- u. Ohrenheilk. (Leipzig) 24, 462–498 (1929)

Dahmann, H.: Zur Physiologie des Hörens II. Ibid. 27, 329–370 (1930)

Dalland, J.: Hearing sensitivity in bats. Science 150, 1185–1186 (1965)

Dice, L., Barto, E.: Ability of mice of the genus Peromyscus to hear ultrasonic sounds. Science 116, 110–111 (1952)

Diercks, K.: Biological sonar systems: a bionics survey. Final Report to the Naval Ship Systems Command. Appl. Res. Lab. Univ. of Texas (Austin), 1–190 (1972)

Dieroff, H. G.: Lärmschwerhörigkeit, Leitfaden der Lärmhörschadenverhütung in der Industrie, München-Berlin-Wien: p. 312 Urban & Schwarzenberg 1975

Doran, A.: Morphology of mammalian Ossicula auditus. Transactions Linn. Soc. London; 2nd ser., 1, Zool. 371–497 (1878)

Elder, J.: Auditory acuity of the chimpanzee. J. Comp. Psychol. 17, 157–183 (1934)

Eschweiler, R.: Zur vergleichenden Anatomie der Muskeln und der Topographie des Mittelohres verschiedener Säugetiere. Arch. mikrosk. Anat. u. Entwicklungsgeschichte (Bonn) 53, 558–622 (1899)

Eysell, A.: Beiträge zur Anatomie des Steigbügels und seiner Verbindungen. Arch. Ohrenheilk. (Würzburg) 5, 237–249 (1870)

Evans, W. E.: Echolocation by marine delphinids and one species of fresh-water dolphin. J. Acoust. Soc. Am. 54, 191–199 (1973)

Feinstein, H.: Acuity of the human sound localization response underwater. J. Acoust. Soc. Am. 53, 393–399 (1973)

Finck, A., Sofouglu, M.: Auditory sensitivity of the mongolian gerbil (Meriones unguiculatus). J. Auditory Res. 6, 313–319 (1966)

Fleischer, G.: Über Schwingungsmessungen am Skelett des Mittelohres von Halicore (Sirenia). Z. Säugetierkunde 36, 350–360 (1971)

Fleischer, G.: Studien am Skelett des Gehörorganes der Säugetiere, einschließlich des Menschen. Säugetierkundl. Mitteilungen (München) 21, 131–239 (1973a)

Fleischer, G.: On structure and function of the middle ear in the bottle-nosed dolphin (Tursiops truncatus). Proc. 9th Annu. Conf. Biol. Sonar and Diving Mammals, pp. 137–179, Menlo Park, Cal.: Stanford Research Inst. 1973b

Fleischer, G.: Structural analysis of the tympanic complex in the bottle-nosed dolphin (Tursiops truncatus). J. Auditory Res. 13, 178–190 (1973c)

Fleischer, G.: On a mechanical model of a bat's middle ear. J. Auditory Res. Suppl. 3, 1–75 (1974)

Fleischer, G.: Über das spezialisierte Gehörorgan von Kogia breviceps (Odontoceti). Z. Säugetierkunde 40, 89–102 (1975)

Fleischer, G.: Hearing in extinct cetaceans as determined by cochlear structure. J. Paleontol. 50, 133–152 (1976a)

Fleischer, G.: Über Beziehungen zwischen Hörvermögen und Schädelbau bei Walen. Säugetierkundl. Mitt. (München) 24, 48–59 (1976b)

Fleischer, G.: Über die Verankerung des Stapes im Ohr der Cetacea und Sirenia. Z. Säugetierkd. 41, 304–317 (1976c)

Fletcher, H., Munson, W.: Loudness, its definition, measurement, and calculation. J. Acoust. Soc. Am. 5, 82–108 (1933)

Francis, R. L.: Behavioural audiometry in mammals: Review and evaluation of techniques. In: Sound reception in mammals, Bench, R., Pye, A., Pye, S. D. (eds.), New York: pp. 237–290, Academic Press 1975

Frank, O.: Die Leitung des Schalles im Ohr. Sitzungsber. der Math. Nat. Kl. Akad. Wiss. (München), 11–77 (1923)

Fraser, F., Purves, P.: Hearing in cetaceans. Bull. Brit. Mus. Nat. Hist.; Zool. 2; 101–114 (1954)

Fraser, F., Purves, P.: Hearing in cetaceans, evolution of the accessory air sacs and the structure and function of the middle ear in recent cetaceans. ibid. 7, 1–140 (1960)

Frey, H.: Vergleichend-anatomische Studien über die Hammer-Amboß Verbindung der Säuger. Anat. Hefte; 1. Abt. (Wiesbaden) 44; 363–437 (1911)

Freye-Zumpfe, H.: Befunde im Mittelohr der Vögel. Wiss. Z., Martin-Luther-Univ. Halle-Wittenberg. Jahrg. 2; (H. 8) Math. Nat. Reihe Nr. 4; 445–461 (1952)

Galambos, R., Rupert, A.: Action of the middle ear muscles in normal cats. J. Acoust. Soc. Am. 31, 349–355 (1959)

Gates, G., Saunders, J., Bock, G.: Peripheral auditory function in the platypus, *Ornithorhynchus anatinus*. J. Acoust. Soc. Am. 56, 152–156 (1974)

Gaupp, E.: Beiträge zur Kenntnis des Unterkiefers der Wirbeltiere I; der Proc. anterior (Folii) des Hammers der Säuger und das Gonial der Nichtsäuger. Anat. Anzeiger (Jena) 39, 97–135 (1911)

Gaupp, E.: Die Reichertsche Theorie (Hammer-, Amboß- und Kieferfrage. Arch. Anat. u. Entwicklungsgeschichte (Leipzig); Suppl.-Band zur Anat. Abt., 1–416 (1912)

Giraud-Sauveur, D.: Recherches biophysiques sur les osselets des cetaces. Mammalia 33; 285–340 (1969)

Glaninger, J.: Untersuchungen zur Festigkeit der Gehörknöchelchen und ihrer Gelenke. Monatsschr. Ohrenheilkd. Laryngo-Rhinol. (Wien) 95, 353–375 (1961)

Goodrich, E. S.: Studies on the Structure and Development of Vertrebrates. Reprinted New York: Dover 1958, p. 837

Griffin, D. R.: Listening in the dark. New Haven: Yale Univ. Press 1958, p. 413

Guinan, J., Peake, W.: Middle-ear characteristics of anesthetized cats. J. Acoust. Soc. Am. 41, 1237–1261 (1967)

Hall, D., Johnson, C.: Auditory thresholds of a killer whale, *Orcinus orca*, L. J. Acoust. Soc. Am. 51, 515–517 (1972)

Hamilton, P.: Underwater hearing thresholds. J. Acoust. Soc. Am. 29, 792–794 (1957)

Hartog, J. P. den: Mechanical vibrations. New York: McGraw-Hill, p. 436 (1956)

Hartridge, H.: Avoidance of obstacles by bats. Nature 156, 55 (1945)

Heezen, B.: Whales entangled in deep sea cables. Deep-Sea Research (Lond.) 4, 105–115 (1957)

Heffner, H., Ravizza, R., Masterton, B.: Hearing in primitive mammals III: Tree shrew (*Tupaia glis*). J. Auditory Res. 9, 12–18 (1969a)

Heffner, H., Ravizza, R., Masterton, B.: Hearing in primitive mammals IV: Bushbaby (*Galago senegalensis*). ibid. 9, 19–23 (1969b)

Heim de Balsac, H.: Les bulles tympaniques des mammifères sahariens; influence du milieu sur leur développment. [Suppl.] Bull. Biol. Fr. Belg. 21, (Paris) 376–408 (1936)

Helmholtz, H.: Die Mechanik der Gehörknöchelchen und des Trommelfells. Arch. ges. Physiol. [Bonn] 1, 1–60 (1868)

Henderson, D., Hamernik, R., Dosanjh, D., Mills, J. (eds.): Effects of Noise on Hearing. New York: Raven Press (1976) p. 565.

Henson, jr., O.: Some morphological and functional aspects of certain structures of the middle ear in bats and insectivores. University of Kansas Sci. Bull. 42 (3), 151–255 (1961)

Hensen, jr., O.: The activity and function of the middle-ear muscles in echo-locating bats. J. Physiol. 180, 871–887 (1965)

Herre, W.: Studien am Skelett des Mittelohres wilder und domestizierter Formen der Gattung *Lama* (Frisch). Acta Anat. (Basel) 19, 271–289 (1953)

Herre, W., Röhrs, M.: Domestikation und Stammesgeschichte. In: Evolution der Organismen. Heberer, G. (ed.), Vol. II/2, pp. 29–151. Stuttgart: Gustav Fischer 1971

Hinchcliffe, R., Pye, A.: Variations in the middle ear of the Mammalia. J. Zool. (London) 157, 277–288 (1969)

Høgmoen, K., Gundersen, T.: Holographic investigation of stapes footplate movements. Acustica 37, 198–202 (1977)

Hollien, H.: Underwater sound localization in humans. J. Acoust. Soc. Am. 53, 1288–1295 (1973)

Hooper, E.: Anatomy of middle-ear walls and cavities in nine species of microtine rodents. Occas. Papers Zool. Museum Michigan (Ann Arbor) 657, 1–28 (1968)

Hyrtl, J.: Vergleichend anatomische Untersuchungen über das innere Gehörorgan des Menschen und der Säugetiere, Prag, p. 150 (1844)

Jacobs, W., Hall, J.: Auditory thresholds of a fresh-water dolphin, *Inia geoffrensis*, Blainville. J. Acoust. Soc. Am. 51, 530–533 (1972)

Johnson, C. S.: Sound detection threshold in marine mammals. In: Marine Bio-Acoustics. Tavolga, W. N. (ed.), Vol. 2. New York: Pergamon 1966, pp. 247–255

Johnson, C. S.: Relation between absolute threshold and duration-of-the-tone pulses in the bottlenosed porpoise. J. Acoust. Soc. Am. 43, 757–763 (1968)

Kasuya, T.: Systematic considerations of recent toothed whales based on the morphology of the tympano-periotic bone. Scient. Repts. Whales Res. Inst. (Tokyo) 25; 1–103

Kartaschew, N., Iljitschow, W.: Über das Gehörorgan der Alkenvögel. J. Ornithol. 105, 113–136 (1964)

Kato, T.: Zur Physiologie der Binnenmuskeln des Ohres. Arch ges. Physiol. (Bonn) 150, 569–625 (1913)

Kellogg, W.: Porpoises and sonar, p. 177. Chicago: Univ. of Chicago Press 1955

Kirikae, I.: Physiology of the middle ear. Arch. Otolaryngology 78; 109–120 (1963)

Klaauw, C. J. van der: The auditory bulla in some fossil mammals. Bull. Amer. Museum of Nat. Hist. 62; 1–352 (1931)

Kobayashi, M.: The articulations of the auditory ossicles and their ligaments of various species of mammalian animals. Hiroshima J. Med. Sci. 4, 319–349 (1955)

Kobrak, H., Lindsay, J., Perlman, H.: Value of the reflex contraction of the muscles of the middle ear as an indicator of hearing. Arch. Otolaryngol. 21, 663–676 (1935)

Kobrak, H.: Construction material of the sound conduction system of the human ear. J. Acoust. Soc. Amer. 20; 125–130 (1948)

Kolmer, W.: Studien am Labyrinth von Insectivoren. Sitzungsber. math.-naturwiss. Kl. Kais. Akad. Wiss. (Wien) 122, 29–52 (1913)

Krebs, B.: Zur frühen Geschichte der Säugetiere. Natur u. Museum (Frankfurt) 105 (5), 147–155 (1975)

Kühne, W. G.: Rhaetische Triconodonten aus Glamorgan, ihre Stellung zwischen den Klassen Reptilia und Mammalia und ihre Bedeutung für die Reichert'sche Theorie. Paläont. Z. 32, 197–235 (1958)

Legouix, J., Petter, F., Wisner, A.: Etude de l'audition des mammifères à bulles tympaniques hypertrophiées. Mammalia 18, 262–271 (1954)

Legouix, J., Wisner, A.: Rôle functionelle des bulles tympaniques géantes de certains rongeurs (Meriones). Acustica 5; 208–216 (1955)

Lindsay, J., Kobrak, H., Perlmann, H.: Relation of the stapedius reflex to hearing sensation in man. Arch. Otolaryngol. 23, 671–678 (1936)

Lorente de No, R., Harris, A.: The threshold of the reflexes of the muscles of the middle ear. Laryngoscope 43, 315–326 (1933)

Lüscher, E.: Die Funktion des M. stapedius des Menschen, I. Zeitschr. f. Hals-, Nasen- u. Ohrenheilkunde (Berlin) 23; 105–132 (1929)

Lüscher, E.: Die Funktion des M. stapedius des Menschen, II. ibid. 25; 462–478 (1930)

McCormick, J., Wever, E., Palin, J., Ridgway, S.: Sound conduction in the dolphin ear. J. Acoust. Soc. Am. 48, 1418–1428 (1970)

McNall, C. L., Chambers, A. H.: Effects of intracochlear pressure changes on cochlear potentials in the guinea pig. J. Auditory Res. 12, 1–7 (1972)

Miller, J. D.: Audibility curve of the chinchilla. J. Acoust. Soc. Am. 48, 513–523 (1970)

Møhl, B.: Hearing in seals. In: The behavior and physiology of pinnipeds, Harrison, R., Hubbard, R., Peterson, R., Rice, C., Schusterman, R. (eds.), pp. 172–195 New York: Meredith Corp. 1968

Møller, A. R.: Transfer functions of the middle ear. J. Acoust. Soc. Am. 35, 1526–1534 (1963)

Møller, A. R.: Function of the middle ear. In: Handbook of Sensory Physiology Vol. V/1, Autrum, H. (ed.), pp. 491–517 Springer 1974a

Møller, A. R.: The acoustic middle ear muscle reflex. ibid. 519–548 (1974b)

Neuweiler, G.: Neurophysiologische Untersuchungen zum Echoortungssystem der Großen Hufeisennase Rhinolophus ferrum equinum Schreber, 1774. Z. vergl. Physiol. 67, 273–306 (1970)

Norris, K. S., Ed.: Whales, Dolphins, and Porpoises. Berkeley and Los Angeles: Univ. of California Press 1966, p. 789

Onchi, Y.: Mechanisms of the middle ear. J. Acoust. Soc. Am. 33, 794–805 (1961)

Payne, R. S., McVay, S.: Songs of humpback whales. Science 173, 585–597 (1971)

Perkins, P. J.: Communication sounds of finnback whales. Norsk Hvalfangst Tidende (Sandefjord) 55, 199–200 (1966)

Peterson, E. A.: Hearing in the lizard: some comments on the auditory capacities of a nonmammalian ear. Herpetologica 22; 161–171 (1966)

64

Peterson, E. A., Wruble, S., Ponzoli, V.: Auditory responses in tree shrews and primates. J. Auditory Res. 8; 345–355 (1968)

Peterson, E. A., Heaton, C., Wruble, S.: Levels of auditory response in fissiped carnivores. J. Mammalogy 50; 566–578 (1969)

Petter, F.: Remarques sur la signification des bulles tympaniques chez les mammifères. Compt Rendu Seanc. Acad. Sc. (Paris) 237, 848–849 (1953)

Pollack, G., Henson, O., Novick, A.: Cochlear microphonic audiograms in the "pure tone" bat Chilonycteris parnelli parnelli. Science 176, 66–68 (1972)

Purves, P. E., Utrecht, W. L. van: The anatomy and function of the ear of the bottle-nosed dolphin (Tursiops truncatus). Beaufortia (Amsterdam) 9; 241–256 (1963)

Purves, P. E.: Anatomy and physiology of the outer and middle ear in cetaceans. pp. 320–380. In: Whales, Dolphins, and Porpoises, Norris, K. S. (ed.), Berkeley, Los Angeles: Univ. of California Press 1966

Pye, A., Hinchcliffe, R.: Structural variations in the mammalian middle ear. Med. Biol. Illus. 18, 122–127 (1968)

Ranke, O. F.: Physiologie des Gehörs. In: Gehör, Stimme, Sprache des Lehrbuches der Physiologie. Trendelenburg, W. u. E., Schütz (eds.), pp. 1–162. Berlin: Springer 1953

Ramprashad, F., Corey, S., Ronald, K.: Anatomy of the seal's ear. In: Functional Anatomy of Marine Mammals. Harrison, R. J. (ed.), Vol. 1, pp. 263–306. London: Academic Press 1972

Reichert, C.: Über die Visceralbogen der Wirbelthiere im Allgemeinen und deren Metamorphosen bei den Vögeln und Säugethieren. Arch. Anat., Physiol. u. wiss. Med. (Leipzig) 120–222 (1837)

Repenning, C.: Underwater hearing in seals: functional morphology. In: Functional Anatomy of Marine Mammals, Vol. 1, Harrison, R. J. (ed.), London: Academic Press 1972 pp. 307–331

Reysenbach de Haan, F. W.: Hearing in whales. Acta Otolaryngol. Suppl. 134, 1–114 (1957)

Robineau, D.: Les osselets de l'ouie de la Rhytine. Mammalia 29, 412–425 (1965)

Robineau, D.: Morphologie externe du complexe osseux temporal chez les siréniens. Mémoirs du Muséum National d'Histoire Naturelle; Nouvelle Série; Série A, Zoologie, 60 (1) 1–32, Paris (1969)

Romer, A.: Cynodont reptile with incipient mammalian jaw articulation. Science 166, 881–882 (1969)

Rubinstein, M., Feldman, B., Fischler, H., Frei, E., Spira, D.: Measurement of stapedial-footplate displacements during transmission of sound through the middle ear. J. Acoust. Soc. Am. 40, 1420–1426 (1968)

Sales, G., Pye, D. (eds.): Ultrasonic communication by animals, p. 281, London: Chapmann and Hall 1974

Schevill, W., Watkins, W., Backus, R.: The 20-cycle signals and Balaenoptera (fin whales). In: Marine Bio-Acoustics, Tavolga, W. N. (ed.), Vol. 1, pp. 147–152. Oxford: Pergamon Press 1964

Schevill, W.: Underwater calls of Trichechus (manatee). Nature 205, 373–374 (1965)

Schwartzkopff, J.: Structure and function of the ear and of the auditory brain areas in birds. In: Ciba Foundation Symposium on Hearing Mechanisms in Vertebrates, Reuck, A. de., Knoght, J. (eds.), pp. 41–59. London: Churchill 1968

Segall, W.: The auditory ossicles (malleus, incus) and their relationships to the tympanic: in Marsupials. Acta Anatomica 73, 176–191 (1969)

Segall, W.: The auditory region (ossicles, sinuses) in gliding mammals and selected representatives of non-gliding genera. Fieldiana Zoology 58; (5), 27–59 (1971)

Segall, W.: Characteristics of the ear, especially the middle ear in fossorial mammals, compared with those in the Manidae. Acta Anatomica 86, 96–110 (1973)

Seilacher, A.: Arbeitskonzept zur Konstruktions-Morphologie. Lethaia (Oslo) 3 (4), 393–396 (1970)

Simmons, F. B.: Perceptual theories of middle ear muscle function. Ann. Otol., Rhinol., Laryngol. 73, 724–739 (1964)

Simmons, F. B.: Binaural summation of the acoustic reflex. J. Acoust. Soc. Amer. 37, 834–836 (1965)

Simmons, J. A.: The sonar receiver of the bat. Annals New York Academy of Science 188, 161–174 (1971)

Smith, J. C.: Sound communication in rodents. In: Sound Reception in Mammals. Bench, R., Pye, A., Pye, S. D. (eds.), pp. 317–330. New York: Academic Press 1975

Solntseva, G. N.: Morpho-functional peculiarities of the hearing organ in terrestrial, semiaquatic, and aquatic mammals. Zool. J. (Moscow) **54**, 1529–1539 (1975)

Starck, D.: Über ein Anlagerungsgelenk zwischen Unterkiefer und Schädelbasis bei den Mausvögeln (Coliidae). Zool. Anzeiger **164**, 1–11 (1960)

Stebbins, W. C.: Hearing of Old World monkeys (*Cercopithecinae*). Amer. J. Phys. Anthrop. **38**; 357–364 (1973)

Stellbogen, E.: Über das äußere und mittlere Ohr des Waldkauzes (*Syrnium aluco, L.*). Z. Morphol. Ökol. Tiere **19**, 686–731 (1930)

Strother, W. F,: Hearing in the chinchilla (*Chinchilla lanigera*): I cochlear potentials. J. Auditory Res. **7**, 145–155 (1967)

Suga, N.: Feature extraction in the auditory system of bats. In: Basic Mechanisms in Hearing. A. Møller (ed.), pp. 675–744. New York; Academic Press 1973

Suga, N., Simmons, J., Jen, P.: Peripheral specialization for fine analysis of Doppler-shifted echoes in the auditory system of the "CF-FM" bat *Pteronotus parnellii*. J. Exp. Biol. **63**, 161–192 (1975)

Tandler, J.: Zur vergleichenden Anatomie der Kopfarterien bei den Mammalia. Denkschr. Kais. Akad. Wiss. (Wien) 1–118 (1898)

Tandler, J.: Zur Entwicklungsgeschichte der Kopfarterien bei den Mammalia. Morphol. Jahrb. (Leipzig) **30**, 275–384 (1902)

Thenius, E.: Stammesgeschichte der Säugetiere (einschließlich der Hominiden). In: Handbuch der Zoologie, Vol. 8, Berlin: (Lief. 47/48) pp. 1–722. De Gruyter 1969

Tonndorf, J.: The role of the tympanic membrane in middle ear transmission. Ann. Otol., Rhinol., Laryngol. **79**, 743–753 (1970)

Tonndorf, J., Khanna, S. M.: Submicroscopic displacement amplitudes of the tympanic membrane (cat) measured by a laser interferometer. J. Acoust. Soc. Am. **44**, 1546–1554 (1968)

Vernon, J.: Hearing in subhuman primates. Primate News (Beaverton) **5**, 5–11 (1967)

Vernon, J., Peterson, E.: Hearing in the vampire bat, *Desmodus rotundus murinus*, as shown by cochlear potentials. J. Auditory Res. **6**, 181–187 (1966)

Vernon, J., Dalland, J., Wever, E.: Further studies of hearing in the bat, *Myotis lucifugus*, by means of cochlear potentials. J. Auditory Res. **6**, 153–163 (1966)

Vernon, J., Herman, P., Peterson, E.: Cochlear potentials in the kangaroo rat, *Dipodomys merriami*. Physiol. Zool. **44**, 112–118 (1971)

Wassif, K.: Anterior process of the malleus in rodents. Nature **157**, 630 (1946)

Wassif, K.: Studies on the structure of the auditory ossicles and tympanic bone in Egyptian Insectivora, Chiroptera and Rodentia. Bull. Faculty of Science, Fouad I Univ. (Cairo) **27**; 177–213 (1948)

Weber, M.: Die Säugetiere, Vol. 1, p. 202. Jena: Fischer 1927

Weber, H.: Stellung und Aufgabe der Morphologie in der Zoologie der Gegenwart. Zool. Anzeiger [Suppl.] **18**, 137–159 (1955)

Webster, D. B.: The ear apparatus of the kangaroo rat, *Dipodomys*. Am. J. Anat. **108**, 123–147 (1961)

Webster, D. B.: A function of the enlarged middle-ear cavities of the kangaroo rat, *Dipodomys*. Physiol. Zool. **35**, 248–255 (1962)

Webster, D. B.: Ear structure and function in modern mammals. American Zoologist **6**; 451–466 (1966)

Wendt, G.: Auditory acuity of monkeys. Comp. Physiol. Monogr. (Baltimore) **10**, 1–51 (1934)

Werner, C. F.: Das Gehörorgan der Wirbeltiere und des Menschen. p. 310. Leipzig: Thieme 1960

Wersäll, R.: The tympanic muscles and their reflexes. Acta Otolaryngol. [Suppl.] **139**, 1–112 (1958)

Wever, E. G., Bray, C. W.: The tensor tympani muscle and its relation to sound conduction. Ann. Otol., Rhinol., Laryngol. **46**, 947–961 (1937)

Wever, E. G., Bray, C. W.: The stapedius muscle in relation to sound conduction. J. Exp. Psychol. **31**, 35–43 (1942)

Wever, E. G., Lawrence, M.: Physiological acoustics, p. 454. Princeton: Princeton Univ. Press 1954

Wever, E. G., Vernon, J. A.: The effects of the tympanic muscle reflexes upon sound transmission. Acta Otolaryngol. **45**, 433–439 (1955)

66

Wever, E. G.: The ear of the Chameleon: *Chamaeleo senegalensis* and *Chamaeleo quilensis*. J. Exp. Zool. **168**, 423–436 (1968)

Wever, E. G., Werner, Y. L.: The function of the middle ear in lizards: *Crotaphytus collaris* (Inguanidae). J. Exp. Zool. **175**, 327–342 (1970)

Winn, H., Perkins, P., Poulter, T.: Sounds of the humpback whale. Proc. 7th Ann. Conf. on Biol. Sonar and Diving Mammals, pp. 39–45 Menlo Park, Cal.: Stanford Research Inst. 1971

Wisner, A., Legouix, J., Petter, F.: Etude histologique de l'oreille d'un rongeur à bulles tympaniques hypertrophiées: *Meriones crassus*. Mammalia **18**, 371–374 (1954)

Wolff, D., Bellucci, R., Eggston, A.: Surgical and Microscopic Anatomy of the Temporal Bone, p. 579. New York: Hafner 1971

Yamada, M.: Contribution to the anatomy of the organ of hearing of whales. Sci. Rep. Whales Res. Inst. (Tokyo) **8**, 1–79 (1953)

Zavattari, E.: Essai d'une interprétation physiologique de l'hypertrophie des bulles tympaniques des Mammifères sahariens. Mammalia **2**, 173–176 (1936)

Zippelius, H., Schleidt, W.: Ultraschall-Laute bei jungen Mäusen. Naturwissenschaften **43**, 502 (1956)

Zwicker, E., Feldtkeller, R.: Das Ohr als Nachrichtenempfänger, p. 232. Stuttgart: Hirzel 1967

Zwislocki, J.: Analysis of the middle-ear function. Part I: Imput impedance. J. Acoust. Soc. Amer. **34**; 1514–1523 (1962)

Zwislocki, J.: Analysis of the middle-ear function. Part II: Guinea-pig ear. ibid. **35**; 1034–1040 (1963)

# Subject Index

# Advances in Anatomy
# Embryology and Cell Biology

# Ergebnisse der Anatomie
# und Entwicklungsgeschichte

# Revues d'anatomie
# et de morphologie expérimentale

*Editors:*
*A. Brodal, Oslo · W. Hild, Galveston · J. van Limborgh, Amsterdam*
*R. Ortmann, Köln · T. H. Schiebler, Würzburg · G. Töndury, Zürich*
*E. Wolff, Paris*

Vol. 55 (Fasc. 1–5)

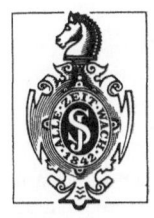

Springer-Verlag Berlin Heidelberg New York 1978

Under § 54 of the German Copyright Law where copies are made for other than private use, a fee is payable to the publishers, the amount of the fee to be determined by agreement with the publishers

ISBN-13: 978-3-540-09140-0                    e-ISBN-13: 978-3-642-67143-2
DOI: 10.1007/978-3-642-67143-2

© Springer-Verlag Berlin Heidelberg 1978

Composition, printing and binding: Universitätsdruckerei H. Stürtz AG, Würzburg

# Contents

# Other Reviews of Interest in this Series

Part 6: **Rohkamm, R.**: Degeneration and Regeneration in Neurons of the Cerebellum. 47 figures. 118 pages. 1977.
ISBN 3-540-08519-X

## Volume 54
Part 1: **Möller, W.**: Circumventriculäre Organe in der Gewebekultur.
34 Abbildungen. 95 Seiten. 1978.
ISBN 3-540-08578-5

Part 2: **Gorgas, K.**: Struktur und Innervation des juxtaglomerulären Apparates der Ratte. 28 Abbildungen. 84 Seiten. 1978.
ISBN 3-540-08615-3

Part 3: **Zilles, K. J.**: Ontogenesis of the Visual System. 43 figures. 138 pages. 1978.
ISBN 3-540-08726-5

Part 4: **Vogel, M.**: Postnatal Development of the Cat's Retina. 27 figures. 66 pages. 1978.
ISBN 3-540-08799-0

Part 5: **Chouchkov, Ch.**: Cutaneous Receptors. 28 figures. 62 pages. 1978.
ISBN 3-540-08826-1

Part 6: **Lüdicke, M.**: Internal Ear Angioarchitectonic of Serpents.
21 figures. 41 pages. 1978.
ISBN 3-540-08836-9

## Volume 55
Part 1: **Reutter, K.**: Taste Organ in the Bullhead (Teleostei).
20 figures. 98 pages. 1978.
ISBN 3-540-08880-6

Part 2: **Dvořák, M.**: The Differentiation of Rat Ova During Cleavage. 62 figures. 131 pages. 1978.
ISBN 3-540-08983-7

Part 3: **Wagner, H.-J.**: Cell Types and Connectivity Patterns in Mosaic Retinas. 30 figures. 81 pages. 1978.
ISBN 3-540-09013-4

Part 4: **Jones, D. G.**: Some Current Concepts of Synaptic Organization. 21 figures. 69 pages. 1978.
ISBN 3-540-09011-8

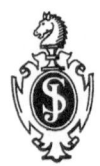

Springer-Verlag Berlin Heidelberg New York